A [...]

with my best regards

Cancer, AIDS, and Quality of Life

Cancer, AIDS, and Quality of Life

Edited by

Jay A. Levy
University of California
San Francisco, California

Claude Jasmin
Hôpital Paul Brousse
Villejuif, France

and

Gabriel Bez
Ministère de la Santé Publique
Paris, France

Plenum Press • New York and London

Library of Congress Cataloging-in-Publication Data

International Council for Global Health Progress. Internationa
  Conference (2nd : 1996 : Paris, France)
    Cancer, AIDS, and quality of life / edited by Jay A. Levy, Claude
  Jasmin, and Gabriel Bez.
       p.   cm.
    "Proceedings of the Second International Conference of the
  International Council for Global Health Progress (ICGHP), held
  January 15-17, 1996, in Paris, France"--T.p. verso.
    Includes bibliographical references and index.
    ISBN 0-306-45517-X
    1. Cancer--Patients--Care--Congresses. 2. AIDS (Disease)-
  -Patients--Care--Congresses. 3. Quality of life--Congresses.
  4. Terminal care--Congresses.   I. Levy, Jay A. II. Jasmin, Claude,
  1938-   . III. Bez, Gabriel. IV. Title.
  RA645.C3I58 1996
  362.1'969792--dc21   97-5782
                                                          CIP

Proceedings of the Second International Conference of the International Council for Global Health
Progress (ICGHP), held January 15 – 17, 1996, in Paris, France

ISBN 0-306-45517-X

© 1997 Plenum Press, New York
A Division of Plenum Publishing Corporation
233 Spring Street, New York, N. Y. 10013

http://www.plenum.com

CONTRIBUTORS

George J. Annas, M.P.H., Professor of Health Law, Schools of Medicine and Public Health, Boston University, Boston, Massachusetts

Mohammed Bedjaoui, President, International Court of Justice, Member, UNESCO Bioethics Committee, The Hague, Netherlands

Robert N. Butler, M.D., Professor of Gerontology and Geriatrics, Director, International Longevity Center, Mount Sinai Medical Center, New York, New York

Daniel Callahan, Ph.D., President, The Hastings Center, Briarcliff Manor, New York

Stephen K. Carter, M.D., Senior Vice-President of Research and Development, Boehringer Ingelheim Pharmaceuticals, Inc., Ridgefield, Connecticut

Robert E. Cawthorn, Chairman of the Board, Rhone-Poulenc Rorer, Inc., Collegeville, Pennsylvania

Paul D. Cleary, Ph.D., Visiting Associate Professor, School of Public Health, Columbia University, New York, New York

Eka Esu-Williams, M.S., Ph.D., AIDSCAP, Calabar, Nigeria

Alvan R. Feinstein, M.D., Professor of Medicine and Epidemiology, School of Medicine, Yale University, New Haven, Connecticut

Harvey V. Fineberg, M.D., Ph.D., Dean, School of Public Health, Harvard University, Boston, Massachusetts

Lieve Fransen, M.D., Ph.D., European Commission, Advisor, Development Cooperation, Brussels, Belgium

Robert J. D. George, M.D., M.R.C.P., Senior Consultant, Palliative Care, University College London, Camden & Islington Community Health Services, National Health Service Trust, London, England

Vassilis Georgoulias, M.D., Professor of Oncology, University of Crete, Director, AIDS National Reference Center of Crete, Crete, Greece

Sonta M. Hunt, Ph.D., Health Research Consultant, London, Founder and Head, European Group for Quality of Life and Health Measurement, London, England

Claude Jasmin, M.D., F.A.C.P., Professor of Oncology, Chairman, Department of Hematology, Immunology and Biology, Hopital Paul Brousse, Villejuif, France

C. R. B. Joyce, Ph.D., FBPsS, Department of Psychology, Royal College of Surgeons, Dublin, Ireland

Jean-Michel Lassaunière, M.D., Palliative Care Team, Hotel Dieu, Paris, France

Jay A. Levy, M.D., Professor, Department of Medicine, Research Associate, Cancer Research Institute, University of California School of Medicine, San Francisco, California

Joanne Lynn, M.D., M.S., Director, Center to Improve the Care of the Dying, George Washington University, Washington, D.C.

Peter Maguire, M.D., Director, Cancer Research Campaign, Psychological Medicine Group, Christie Hospital, Manchester, England

Joan Marks, Director, Graduate Programs in Human Genetics and Health Advocacy, Sarah Lawrence College, Bronxville, New York

Paul A. Marks, M.D., Ph.D., President, Memorial Sloan-Kettering Cancer Center, New York, New York

M. Federico Mayor, Director General, UNESCO, Paris, France

John Orley, M.D., M.R.C.P., Senior Medical Officer, Mental Health Promotion, Program on Mental Health, World Health Organization, Geneva, Switzerland

Patrice Pinell, M.D., Director, INSERM U158, University Rene Descartes, Paris, France

Peter Piot, M.D., Director, Division of Research and Intervention Development, Global Program on AIDS, World Health Organization, Geneva, Switzerland

Joan Rovira, Ph.D., Department of Economics, University of Barcelona, Research Director, SOIKOS, S.L., Center for Applied Studies in Health Economics and Social Policy, Barcelona, Spain

Lisbeth Sachs, Ph.D., Department of International Health and Social Medicine, Unit of International Health Care Research, Karolinska Institute, Stockholm, Sweden

Ibrahim M. Shoaib, M.D., Professor, Faculty of Medicine, Tanta University, Tanta, Egypt

Robert A. Zittoun, M.D., Professor and Chairman, Department of Hematology, Hotel-Dieu, Paris, France

PREFACE

This volume contains selected contributions from individuals who attended the Second International Conference of the International Council for Global Health Progress (ICGHP) held at UNESCO in Paris, France, on January 15–17, 1996. This conference brought together experts in many disciplines that deal with the devastating diseases of cancer and AIDS with a focus on the concerns for quality of life. The ICGHP fosters multicultural and, multidisciplinary approaches to global health problems to help influence governments and other international health organizations to emphasize prevention and care of diseases and to understand their scientific, social, and cultural features. The Council encourages the interchange of information on health problems and policy and supports educational funding for the public at large. Its objective is to effect diseases-free lives in the world community.

Participants of the conference included scientists, sociologists, government leaders, physicians, health care providers, epidemiologists, religious leaders, company officials, ethicists, and philosophers. They examined and discussed the many variables involved in quality of life for people affected with cancer and with AIDS. The volume's text begins with introductory comments by officials attending the ICGHP conference. Subsequently, a chapter is dedicated to one aspect of quality of life, be it definition, scientific research, evolution, cultural changes, ethics, measurements, or other issues dealing with health care and treatment survival.

The second part of the volume includes commentaries dealing with five aspects of quality of life which merit consideration. It is the hope of the Council and the participants of this conference that the contributions presented in this volume will help define further the importance of quality of life in dealing with any illness, but particularly with cancer and with AIDS. These diseases affect not only the patient but the patient's family, the community, and the doctor/patient relationship. All of these participants in health care delivery need to be considered in the final approaches at bringing the best quality of life to the individual.

Jay A. Levy, M.D.
San Francisco
Claude Jasmin, M.D.
Paris
Gabriel Bez
Paris

ACKNOWLEDGMENTS

The Second International Conference was held under the auspices of the President of France, Jacques Chirac, the President of the European Commission, Jacques Santer, and the Director General of UNESCO, Federico Mayor. The volume's editors would like to acknowledge the patronage of the following: The French Ministry of Public Health; Mr. Philippe Douste Blazy, Minister of Culture; the European Academy of Arts, Sciences, and Humanities; UNAIDS; INSERM (National Institute of Health and Medical Research); ANRS (National Agency for AIDS Research); Assistance Publique, Hopitaux de Paris; Faculty of Medicine Paris Sud, University Paris XI; Foundation de France; and the IUCC (International Union Against Cancer). The Conference was substantially supported by contributions from the following organizations: Commission Europeenne, Foundation de France, Foundation Goldsmith, Syndicat National de l'Industrie Pharmaceutique, Bristol-Myers Squibb, Lafon, Rhone-Poulenc Rorer Foundation, Roche, Sandoz, Sanofi Winthrop, Synthelabo, and Theramex. Moreover, we acknowledge the support of Amgen, Janssen-Cilag, Wyeth-Lederle, Pharmacia and Upjohn, and Shering-Plough. We also thank Asta Medica, Chiron (France), Ernst & Young International, Glaxo Wellcome, Journal du SIDA, Lavoisier Abonnements, Institut Lilly, Leo Research Foundation, Leo (France), Mapi Research Institute, Pierre Fabre Medicament, Cabinet Reussites - Resources Humaines, Regimedia S.A., Servier, Societe Française de Lymphologie, and Zeneca Pharma for their help with the Conference. Finally, the editors would like to thank Dr. Peter Berczeller and Christine Beglinger for their help in the preparation of this volume and acknowledge the assistance of the Coordinating Committee: Regine Boutrais, Catherine Guyot, Michele Liegeon, Catherine Toesca, and Rebecca Bokhobza.

CONTENTS

INTRODUCTION

Cancer and AIDS as a Model for the Study of Quality of Life 1
    Claude Jasmin

United Nations Educational, Scientific, and Cultural Organization 5
    M. Federico Mayor

Joint United Nations Program on HIV/AIDS (UNAIDS) 7
    Peter Piot

CANCER, AIDS, AND QUALITY OF LIFE

1. Problems in Defining Quality of Life 11
    Alvan R. Feinstein

2. How Does Basic Research in Cancer and AIDS Approach the Concern for
        Quality of Life? 17
    Jay A. Levy

3. The Evolution of Quality of Life 37
    C. R. B. Joyce

4. Quality of Care for Cancer and AIDS 45
    Robert J. D. George

5. Changing Our Metaphors to Put Quality of Life at the Center of Health Care . . . 55
    George J. Annas

6. Uses of Information about Health-Related Quality of Life in Patients with AIDS
        and Cancer 63
    Paul D. Cleary

7. Improving the Quality of Life of Cancer Patients 73
    Peter Maguire

8. How Does the Cost of Care Influence the Effectiveness of Health Care Delivery?   77
    Joan Rovira and Patricia Alegre

9. Future Issues in the Use of Health Status Assessment Measures in Clinical
        Settings   85
    Sheldon Greenfield, Sherrie H. Kaplan, and Ira B. Wilson

10. Quality of Life at the End Stages of Life   89
    Daniel Callahan

COMMENTARIES

A. Quality of Life: Who Is Responsible?

11. Quality of Life: The Experience of an Oncology Unit Functioning in a Rural
        Greek Area   97
    Vassilis Georgoulias, Charalaubos Kourousis, and Stelios Kakolyris

12. Advocacy for Patients with Cancer Quality of Life Implications   101
    Joan Marks

B. Quality of Life: Who Defines It?

13. Risk as Diagnosis: Implications for the Quality of Life   107
    Lisbeth Sachs

14. Quality of Life as a Major Determinant of Medical Decision-Making   115
    Robert Zittoun

C. Quality of Life at the End Stages of Life

15. Quality of Life at the End Stages of Life   119
    Mohammed Bedjaoui

16. Cancer, AIDS, and Quality of Life   129
    Robert N. Butler

17. Anguish and Suffering in the Face of the Hospital Organizational Pattern   131
    Jean-Michel Lassaunière

18. Living Well in the Shadow of Death   137
    Joanne Lynn

D. Quality of Life: Socio-Economic, Geographic, and Cultural Factors

19. Quality of Life: Cultural, Socio-Economic, and Geographic Perspectives   141
    Eka Esu-Williams

20. Quality of Life: Socio-Economic, Geographic, and Cultural Factors   147
    Lieve Fransen

21. Quality of Life: An Unsuitable Case for Measurement?   155
    Sonta M. Hunt

22. Quality of Life: Geographic and Cultural Differences   159
    John Orley

23. Cancer and Quality of Life: Social and Community Stakes   163
    Patrice Pinell

24. The HIV/AIDS Epidemic in Developing Countries: The Dilemma of Quality of
    Life vs Quality of Care   169
    Ibrahim M. Shoaib

E. Quality of Life: Pharmaceutical Considerations

25. Quality of Life: Some Implications of the Advances in Human Genome Research   173
    Paul A. Marks

26. Quality of Life in Cancer and AIDS: An Industry Perspective   179
    Stephen K. Carter

27. Quality of Life, Value, and Price in Medicines to Treat Serious Disease   183
    Robert E. Cawthorn

Conclusion   189
    Harvey V. Fineberg

Index   193

CANCER AND AIDS AS A MODEL FOR THE STUDY OF QUALITY OF LIFE

Claude Jasmin

President of the International Council for Global Health Progress
Hospital Paul Brousse
14. av. Paul Vaillant Couturier
94807 Villejuif Cedex
France

I. QUALITY OF LIFE AND CARE

Cancer is often a debilitating and painful example of an archetypal chronic illness. Its spontaneous evolution and its treatments are well known to substantially affect the personal, family and social life of the patient. This fact explains the significant development in the measures taken to integrate Quality of Life into the treatment of cancer.

AIDS is also a chronic process. Today AIDS is still an incurable disease, and the mean duration of life of patients after diagnosis is often equal or superior to 10 years.

Cancer and AIDS symbolize the hopes and disappointments of the medical revolution of the 20th century. Thus, despite the great progress made in the cancer biology field, the average rate of recovery from cancer does not exceed 50%. On the other hand, the AIDS outbreak reminds us that infectious risks are far from being eliminated and that new viral diseases can and do endanger the health of the world.

The demands of patients and their families for taking quality of life into account and the recent interest of doctors in measuring quality of life have appeared in reaction to the current limits on the possibilities for recovery from these two diseases.

This congress will compare cancer and AIDS in studying Quality of Life as a new measuring tool for the results of medical therapeutic intervention on the one hand, and as a concept for increasing our knowledge of the new social situation engendered by these terrible diseases in the last 25 years on the other.

The AIDS upsurge has overturned the relationship between patients, doctors and society. As a matter of fact, patients infected with the HIV virus have united into an active and powerful group which heads the struggle to "lead one's disease time". The traditional attitude of patients with cancer is generally passive, whereas that of patients with AIDS is strong and confrontational, especially in the developed countries. This activism has had important effects in public health care management.

Cancer, AIDS, and Quality of Life, edited by Levy *et al.*
Plenum Press, New York, 1997

The social repercussions of cancer and AIDS have stimulated significant consequences in several research fields:

  a. The search for new treatments based on the major progress made in the last ten
     years in the understanding of these two diseases: the use of cytokines, gene ther-
     apy and development of new anti-cancer drugs. In the AIDS sector, we have
     seen both the development of antiviral chemotherapy, previously not of great in-
     terest, and of intensive research into the definitive version of an HIV vaccine.
  b. The development of care facilities which are more flexible, and also adaptable
     to the preservation of a better family and social environment for the patients:
     hospital community cooperative ventures associating hospital doctors with local
     doctors within care networks in which patients have an important role; accep-
     tance of a joint effort between associations of AIDS patients and care deciders
     with the aim of innovating the organization of patient care. This tendency is
     much more striking in the case of AIDS than that of cancer, since patients with
     cancer are treated at the hospital during the day, benefit from ambulatory and
     home care, and are not able to control the care channels managed by powerful
     hospital-based teams.

On the other hand, it is in the care of patients with terminal cancer that palliative
care units have been established in the developed countries. These exist in order to remedy
the situation in the terminal phase where care deciders such as doctors, psychologists, and
nurses face a feeling of professional failure.

These days, as a matter of fact, doctors are not prepared to care for patients when technical means for struggling against disease turn out to be ineffective. Instead they are confronted with a sense of professional failure which paralyzes them: patients' Quality of Life
appears to them to be an illusory objective; at bottom they do not know how to overcome the
physical and moral pain of their patient. Moreover, they underestimate the level of pain as is
shown in a study performed by the Pain Society of Great Britain, which is still in the experimental phase of palliative care. According to this study, one third of the 160 000 people dying
of cancer every year in that country did not receive appropriate treatment for their pain1 !

In other words, care deciders cannot accept failure, but at the same time they are not
prepared to deal with either physical or psychic pain. Optimism brought on by medical
progress keeps doctors from hearing what Emmanuel Levinas had to say about a medical
"vocation": "In suffering, there is a cry and a sigh, a moan. It is the first prayer. It is the
origin of prayer; words addressed to the absent. The doctor is the one who hears these
moans. As a result, the initial response to this plea for help may well be a medical one,
and this symbolizes the medical calling of man". It is in this context that Quality of Life
assumes importance as a possible tool of medical progress better adapted to patient needs.

II. MEASURING QUALITY OF LIFE, A RESEARCH TOOL

The definition of Quality of Life functions in conjunction with the definition of
health by the WHO. Its aim is to measure as much as possible the perception by the patient of his somatic, emotional and social well-being. In this way, Quality of Life functions as the interface between medicine and research in psychology.

Although criticism abounds regarding the validity of the methods in use, and despite
a great diversity of models and scales of Quality of Life, a consensus appears to be in

place regarding utilization of Quality of Life measures in the estimation of outcome of care in patients afflicted with cancer or AIDS.

A recently published study shows that "cancer patients' reporting of somatic symptoms by means of a standardized Quality of Life questionnaire is closely related to emotional and social distress, and is not equivalent to health status as determined from a clinical perspective"[2].

In addition, this study points to the importance of negative affect on the well-being of patients, and "deserves attention as an important signal for intervention in follow-up programs of tumors".

Quality of Life can be useful to care deciders, particularly doctors, so as to improve their perception of how patients experience their illness, and the interaction between the patient and his social and familial environment.

Quality of Life has become an important criterion in the area of drug research. It is the function of drug companies to tie the therapeutic advantage of a molecule to gain for the patient. This concern for the comfort of the patient has, in the past 10 years, manifested itself in the ever growing number of articles dedicated to this theme.

Furthermore, measurement of Quality of Life has been accepted as a criterion for approval of marketing of new drugs by national and international drug agencies. During a drug trial, it is no longer sufficient to answer questions such as: "Is it safe?" or "How effective is it?" Nowadays we have to respond to at least two other questions: "What does this drug do for the Quality of the patient's Life?" and: "What is the cost - benefit ratio in terms of Quality of Life?".

The notion of quality of life thus becomes a subject that must be addressed when the economic aspects of health are considered.

The notable association of patients stricken with AIDS and their national political representatives, (particularly as regards medications), and their tense, sometimes violent dialogue with representatives of the pharmaceutical industry, provide evidence of this confrontativeness on the political level. Far from being opposed to this social right of patients' associations, the pharmaceutical industry is attempting to define areas of common interest for both parties.

III. QUALITY OF LIFE IN THE MIDST OF A SOCIAL DEBATE IN THE DEVELOPED COUNTRIES

Examination of the Quality of Life of patients who suffer from cancer or AIDS pulls us into a social and philosophical debate characteristic of our new medicine. By virtue of its effectiveness and its practical applications, biological research has turned around the traditional side of medicine. For instance this happens in the time-space aspect of sickness, when a simple blood test makes it possible today to detect infection with the HIV virus which will however manifest itself clinically much later or possibly even never.

In the same way today, molecular biology makes it possible to discover, starting with the intra-uterine stage, the mutations of certain chromosomes which predispose to several types of cancers.

Indeed, classical microbiology and traditional genetics can in some cases predict the risk of infectious or hereditary diseases. But technological progress in biology in the last 10 years has been widening the range of pre-clinical detection of multiple diseases: infections, cancers, so-called degenerative diseases...

Potential consequences of this technological progress in terms of Quality of Life are multiple and complicated. They pose new ethical and socio-economical problems.

For instance, widespread distribution of genetic predictive tests of potentially serious diseases could provoke the emergence of a category of patients which I like to call genopositive, in other words, those who are liable to become a pressure group such as did HIV seropositives. Care deciders such as doctors and nurses are not prepared for a new medical situation which a large group of high-risk individuals would represent, one whose somatic and psychological care must be assumed both on the individual and family level. It is perhaps thanks to the detection that researchers will discover new preventive therapeutic methods. Yet the question in this case is still how to manage the costs of long massive, multiple studies with uncertain outcome. Even the simple medical care of these high-risk families could turn out to be a heavy economic burden for the countries liable to disseminate these tests. In this way, technology linked to this sudden expansion of the medical sphere, could put at risk the social protection against disease considered an inalienable right in most developed countries.

Yet, going beyond the difficult and almost unbearable problem involved in making choices arising from an economical and political vision of health, the heart of the debate concerns the aims for and the medical philosophy of the 21th century. The question is how it will resolve the dilema which arises from the expansion of the demand for medical services which comes from modern man, especially in Western countries. This applies to those who suffer from illnesses in their traditional definition and those who have a wish for improvement without having a real illness. Without clearly defined limits, medical social or economic, these needs will never be satisfied... In parallel to this need to control disease and pain, the euthanasia ideology is gaining ground in Europe and in the United States based on the perceived right to dispose of one's life as well as one's body.

Quality of Life thus could well be in the midle of an ideological, philosophical and deontological confrontation, and of utilitarian choices recommended by the economists in the name of a fair division of the resources which are limited even for the richest countries.

What can be said of the Quality of Life of the people in developing countries? How can they benefit from these debates led by rich countries? What can they teach us that is essential, if not the fragility of the human condition and the socio-economic and sanitary inequality which abounds on our planet?

The debate opened by this congress is important and must be extended beyond its duration. If cancer and AIDS symbolize especially important examples, because they are universally recorded on people's imaginations, whatever their geographical origins or their philosophical convictions or their socio-economic situations, this congress aims at emphasizing the importance of Quality of Life as a measuring tool for medical activity. Will this new tool be useful in once more placing the Western doctor into a more comprehensive relationship with his patient, by clarifying certain psychological needs neglected heretofore by "scientific" medicine?

The exceptional quality of the participants of this congress and its site, a symbol of universal culture, give me confidence in the benefits that all those in attendance will gather whatever their discipline or origins.

REFERENCES

1. Mentioned by the Agence Presse Medicale, France, April 1996.
2. Koller M., Kussman J., Lorenz W. Etal: Symptom Reporting in Cancer Patients:the Role of Negative Affect and Experienced Social Trauma Cancer. vol. 77, 983–995, 1996.

UNITED NATIONS EDUCATIONAL, SCIENTIFIC, AND CULTURAL ORGANIZATION

M. Federico Mayor

Director General
UNESCO
7 place de Fontenoy
75532 Paris, France

We are very pleased to welcome you to UNESCO, this house of all cultures, and we would like to express how much we appreciate your giving us the summary of your reflections on a number of essential issues dealing with the present and the future of the human community.

I have been following the various religious and cultural approaches - Protestant, Buddhist, Catholic, Jewish, Muslim - and they confirm my own view that quality of life in a democratic system cannot be expressed in terms of a privileged elite. Quality of life depends on all the elements of society - not only on civil society, as is very often said. Religious representatives and military forces must today more than ever - particularly on the eve of a new century - be seen to make their contribution to the quality of life. Quality of life - particularly in those dispersed human settlements, in rural areas, where there is exclusion and asymmetry - requires a frame-work of caring and of sharing.

I am particularly worried about the immense disparities that exist in the distribution of wealth and the many other kinds of sharing, particularly regarding gender disadvantage. In a world in which at least 95% of the power and decision-making is in the hands of men, and only 4–5% belonging to women, in a world in which certain citizens and the citizens of certain countries possess 80% of all resources, quality of life cannot exist. While health is important, dignity is even more important. Dignity cannot exist in a context of immense imbalances. I am, therefore, glad to hear it emphasized that every single person counts. This is democracy.

Democracy does not consist of being counted in public opinion polls or in elections every three or four or five years; democracy means that we all count as citizens. Democracy often takes into account the macro approach which does not concern itself with aspects at the level of the individual. We must start to think in terms of micro patterns, and to operate at the level of the everyday life of the individual. Then, and only then, can we reach the quality of life, because we will then be dealing with the sharing of wealth, health and decision-making.

Cancer, AIDS, and Quality of Life, edited by Levy *et al.*
Plenum Press, New York, 1997

There is a point in common between those involved in AIDS research and UNESCO: we both aim at prevention. The United Nations system is entrusted with maintaining peace; but, when all is said and done, peace-keeping operations are implying failure. It is after the conflict, after the suffering and the destruction that the blue berets intervene. As a matter of fact, priority should be given to the prevention of conflicts. Prevention means to see as well as to foresee; it dignifies vigilantes, anticipation of problems and recommends intervention, before differences are exaggerated. Just as a doctor detects the precursory sign of an illness, so we should aim at the early detection of crises.

The topic at this conference concerns all of us since it deals with safeguarding the quality of our own lives and maintaining, as far as possible, that of the ill. The growing concern for the quality of life can, to some extent, be explained by scientific progress which allows life to be prolonged. However, the effects of science can sometimes be quantitative rather than qualitative, and this gives rise to further questioning and review.

UNESCO shares many of the concerns that are being expressed. Examples include the need to focus strategies of quality of life on the patient and bring attention to the obligation of the doctor to 'accompany' the patient (without getting ahead of him), and the duty to keep the patient informed, within limits, while maintaining his dignity and integrity.

You also raise the question of the ways of measuring quality of life. It has been said that quality of life is subjective - as much a state of mind as a state of health. This may be so, but is not the objective/subjective dialectic somewhat artificial? As the great Spanish poet, Jose Bergamin, said, there are as many subjective ideas as there are subjects, and objectivity belongs only to the object. It is obvious that quality of life and health are intimately related. The important thing is to confer a certain quality of life on the sick.

In conclusion, allow me to come back to prevention. From my years as a biochemist working on the pathology of the brain of newborn infants, I maintain a firm conviction of the vital need for prevention, but at the same time an awareness of its invisibility. Prevention is invisible because it prevents the manifestation of pathology; it is invisible as is health. In this respect, it is not "newsworthy." It is up to us to underscore the every day, the "normal", the healthy, the intangible - so discreet and yet so essential.

As you know, UNESCO is involved in preventive education. It is involved with other institutions and United Nations agencies in forming a broad front against the AIDS epidemic, which is so much more than just a health problem. Only if we act together, in concert, at national and international, governmental and non-governmental levels, in laboratories and the field, will we be able to fully recognize the challenge and at last find a solution. Until this remedy is found, we must concentrate on the dignity and integrity of the patient, two qualities which themselves alone are at the very foundation of human solidarity.

JOINT UNITED NATIONS PROGRAM ON HIV/AIDS (UNAIDS)

Peter Piot

ONUSIDA
OMS
CH-1211 Geneve 27 Suisse

INTRODUCTION

In my comments on quality of life, I would like particularly to stress the needs generated by AIDS in developing countries. There, like everywhere else, AIDS is a fatal and often unmentionable disease. There, like everywhere else, we still haven't found a cure or a vaccine. There, like everywhere else, it is an epidemic that strikes people at the most productive age.

What is unique in the Third World is the scale of the problem. Nine out of ten people are seropositive. There, almost 6,000 people are infected *every day.* And that is among the poorest of people. Of course, quality of life doesn't just depend on medical care. Fortunately. But care is essential all the same. And there, resources are desperately short.

The problem is only just beginning. We reckon that there are over a million people with AIDS in developing countries today, and that could easily double before we reach the year 2000. Don't forget the millions of people who are seropositive, including those who are unaware of it, who could really benefit from advice and voluntary testing. We can't talk about AIDS without mentioning the needs of the relatives of AIDS victims, the partners, the elderly parents, the orphans affected by the epidemic. They need care, admittedly a different kind of care, but care that is essential for their quality of life.

THE JOINT UNITED NATIONS PROGRAM ON AIDS

(UNAIDS) came fully into being just two weeks ago. We are a small joint venture cosponsored by six organizations in the United Nations family. Our cosponsors have complementary mandates and strengths ranging from development to health, from education to family planning. UNAIDS was born of the recognition that the causes and consequences

Cancer, AIDS, and Quality of Life, edited by Levy *et al.*
Plenum Press, New York, 1997

of AIDS cut across sectoral lines - they include health but go far beyond it. So our mission is to lead an expanded response to the epidemic.

Many are well aware that in the field of AIDS, international concern has been dominated up to now by prevention. AIDS care has had a lower priority - some might call it the poor relation - *le parent pauvre*. UNAIDS aims to turn this situation around. Care in the broadest sense is going to receive equal billing with prevention. Enhancing the quality of life will be a major focus of our efforts in advocacy, work with countries and research.

What do we at UNAIDS mean by "quality of life"? According to our working definition, quality of life is an individual's perception of his or her position in life - in the context of the local culture and value systems, and in relation to the individual's own goals, expectations and concerns. "Quality of life" is thus defined **by** the person. And it embraces many dimensions, including the physical and psychological domains, level of independence, social relationships, the person's environment, and the spiritual domain.

MAXIMIZING QUALITY OF LIFE IN THE AIDS ERA

I come now to the issue of what needs to be done to improve quality of life in the AIDS era. It is tempting to set out a very long list here, but I will try to outline just five areas of need whichshould be concidered.

1. Respect

The first area is that of respect for people living with or affected by HIV - respect for their human rights and their human dignity. It is inadmissible that AIDS continues to elicit discrimination, hostility and rejection, even in parts of the world that have had plenty of time to come to terms with this epidemic. Treating people humanely is bound to improve their quality of life in at least four of the dimensions I mentioned earlier. And humane treatment is affordable - it carries no price tag. It should be just as accessible in poor settings as in rich ones.

By the way, one means of respecting people with HIV is to ensure that they are active participants in planning and organizing their own care. Our broad definition of quality of life makes it clear that they are the best placed to determine what they need.

2. Psychological Support

The second area of need is for psychological support, under which I include voluntary counselling and testing, or VCT. In the international arena VCT has not received much emphasis - partly because of concerns about its cost, but also because of fear of inadvertently encouraging the proponents of mandatory testing. HIV testing is a complex issue in which there are no easy answers, but I feel it is time for the pendulum to swing towards VCT. It is a human right to know one's serostatus if one so wishes. People can not get the support or care they need, or plan for themselves or their survivors, if they don't know they are infected.

VCT services offer broader public health benefits too. VCT can help break through the conspiracy of silence that surrounds the presence of HIV in a family or community. Trained counsellors can help clients to balance their need for confidentiality with their need to inform and get support from close family members.

3. Palliative Care

Respect and support are essential for quality of life - but they are not sufficient. Less than a month ago, while I was in Uganda for the International Conference on AIDS, I visited a centre in Kampala run by the AIDS service organization known as TASO. This non-goverment organization (NGO) provides impressive counselling and social support to over 200 000 Ugandans living with HIV. In fact, TASO has played a pioneering role in this domain in Africa and, indeed, in the world.

I had the privilege of speaking with dozens of patients whom I found really sophisticated in their understanding of AIDS - just like AIDS patients in Europe. They knew so much, but, apart from counselling, they had so little to ease their suffering.

The fact is that thousands of patients in the developing world are living with and dying from AIDS without so much as an aspirin to ease their misery. A recent study in Kenya showed that around 30% of AIDS patients die without ever coming into contact with the formal health system. Which brings me to the third area of need - palliative care. It is a scandal that a person with severe headache lacks even a simple analgesic, that children have to watch their sick parents scratch themselves till they're bloody, or that a family caring for an AIDS patient with diarrhoea can not even afford a bar of soap.

But people with AIDS are not the only ones in need. Those suffering from intolerable pain and discomfort because of cancer and other conditions have just as great a claim to palliation. And this is a claim that is increasingly being acknowledged *outside* the health sphere, too. For example, the **World Development Report** published by the World Bank - one of our six cosponsors - recommends that pain relief should be part of the so-called essential care package made available even in the poorest countries.

We calculate that with ten or so simple items - including soap - we could minimize the suffering from itching, nausea, diarrhoea, thrush and headache, whether associated with AIDS or another condition. No sophisticated clinical studies are needed here - what we must have is political leadership and some simple operational research.

4. Prophylaxis and Treatment

The fourth area of need I want to highlight is treatment. Not sophisticated treatment with antiretrovirals - for most people in the developing world, this is unlikely to become accessible at any time soon. No, I am talking about prophylaxis and treatment for the common opportunistic infections, which are vital to maintaining a tolerable quality of life.

It has become standard, although not universal practice in the developed world, to undertake the prevention of some opportunistic infections and not wait for actual episodes of illness. Now it is becoming clear that this approach is both feasible and cost-effective in the developing countries too. Research is showing us the way. For example, a picture of effectiveness is beginning to emerge from research on prophylaxis of tuberculosis. And TB prophylaxis has been estimated to cost just $14 a year - less than for treating episodes of TB as they occur. Can we really call this unaffordable?

Prophylaxis for bacterial pneumonia, toxoplasmosis and septicaemia may also be feasible and cost-effective. With our support, two studies on these are about to start in South Africa and Malawi. Practical clinical research of this kind will be a major priority for UNAIDS.

5. Family Support

The fifth and final area of need is for family support. The needs are very great indeed in the case of AIDS, which clusters in families as first one and then both parents become infected.

AIDS orphans number in the millions. In many hard-hit communities they have overwhelmed the coping capacity of the extended family, as uncles and aunts die leaving only elderly grandparents to care for a dozen or more youngsters. By any yardstick, the quality of life of AIDS orphans is often abysmal.

Even *before* their parents die, children suffer one loss after the other as family income drops, parental care falters, and the child ren themselves wind up taking care of the very adults who would normally be taking care of them. Girls in particular are often taken out of school to help shoulder the burden of care, which generally falls on the women of the family - who are often ill themselves.

Only through a fairer sharing of the care burden by men and women, and through more community and external support for affected families and survivors, can we hope to improve their quality of life.

CONCLUSION

In conclusion, neither cancer nor AIDS nor cancer can be considered in isolation from other ills and problems, and especially not in isolation from the general state of health of our society. If we are to ensure a better quality of life, we need remedies that range from more respect for human rights through equality for women to better pay for health workers.

What about the issue of health care financing? Here, the prime need is to take a critical look at how the vast sums now being spent are allocated. I venture to say there is considerable misspending both public and private. For example, government expenditure on sophisticated hospitals absorbs much of the total health budget in some developing countries at the same time that primary health care goes begging. And individuals spend vast amounts on useless remedies instead of the simple medicines for pain and itching they really need.

So I am not averse to the reform movement sweeping the world. Health care financing *does* need scrutiny and reform. But even more than a balanced budget, we should be striving for a balanced and better use of our health resources. If we are serious about ensuring a decent quality of life for all, reorienting public and private expenditure is a moral imperative.

1

PROBLEMS IN DEFINING QUALITY OF LIFE

Alvan R. Feinstein

Yale University School of Medicine
New Haven, Connecticut

The main goal of my remarks is to point out the problems of the customary approach, commonly used in clinical trials and other studies of therapy, that measures "quality of life" as though it were a state of health. With this approach, quality of life is expressed as the sum of ratings for a series of domains referring to symptoms, physical functions, and other components of "health".

STATE OF THE MIND VS. STATE OF HEALTH

Perhaps the main flaw of this strategy is that quality of life is a state of mind, not a state of health[1]. Individual persons appraise their quality of life as reflecting feelings of well-being and other subjective, personal reactions to their state of health and to many other non-medical features of life. These features can include family relationships, social and occupational activities, spirituality, creativity, economic security, resilience, hopes, disappointments, fears, joys, and sorrows. These non-medical features of human existence may make certain patients feel they have an excellent quality of life despite major physical disability. Conversely, other patients may have poor quality of life despite being in an excellent state of health. Consequently, quality of life cannot be adequately appraised with indexes (or other measurements) that concentrate on health status.

A second flaw is the custom of expressing quality of life as a rating in an index whose components are determined, weighted, and combined according to statistical principles that reflect the beliefs and decisions of various experts or academic authorities. The problem here is that a patient's well-being or state of mind can be expressed only by the patient, or perhaps by family or friends who are close enough to know the patient's state of mind. The patient's own beliefs cannot be suitably indicated by an expert's rating of health status. Furthermore, when that rating is obtained by mathematically summing a set of component ratings for individual variables, an undesirable new phenomenon is produced: statistical reductionism.

Cancer, AIDS, and Quality of Life, edited by Levy *et al.*
Plenum Press, New York, 1997

CONCEPTS OF REDUCTIONISM

A hallmark of 20th Century biologic science has been the strategy of reductionism. One feature of the reductionist approach is to replace a complex phenomenon with a simpler model. Thus, we may study animals rather than people, or more elementary organisms, such as paramecia, rather than rats. A second feature of reductionism is the decomposition of a whole into its component parts. Thus, we may study organs such as the liver or kidney, instead of studying an intact person. Organs may be further reduced to tissues, tissues to cells, and cells to molecules.

The reductionist strategy began in 19th Century science, and was intended to explain the mechanisms of phenomena that occur in nature and disease. The strategy has been excellent and magnificently successful in leading to our modern scientific advances in knowledge of pathophysiology and molecular biology. The strategy has also led to development of some of the splendid technologic procedures that are used in modern medical diagnosis and therapy.

Biologic reductionism has been heavily criticized, however, because medical scientists have been distracted from contemplating what happens to intact people, and also because the reductionist approach does not observe and therefore cannot appraise symptoms, functional capacity, or the mental and psychic status of intact persons. The additional difficulties are that a simpler model may distort, disguise, or evade the reality that occurs in the more complex organism. For example, we do not discuss quality of life for a rat or for a kidney, although we might be able to measure the corresponding state of health. In addition, a whole may not be merely a sum of the parts. For example, if we take a clock apart and examine its wheels, gears, and springs, we may get an excellent idea of how the clock works but only in the intact clock can we determine whether it tells time correctly.

STATISTICAL REDUCTIONISM

An extraordinary irony of the current medical scene is that complaints of intact patients being ignored during biologic reductionism are now apparently being solved by introducing statistical reductionism. In one form of statistical reductionism, we take the complex clinical spectrum of a disease and replace it by compression into the results for an "average" patient. This type of reductionism constantly occurs in randomized statistical trials of therapy. In a second form of statistical reductionism, meaningful clusters of categories in biologic thinking — such as congestive heart failure, widely metastatic cancer, or pancytopenia — are replaced by algebraic linear models[2] that combine the components not in categorical clusters, but in a sum of weighted variables such as

$$Y = b_0 + b_1 X_1 + b_2 X_2 + b_3 X_3 + \dots .$$

The third form of statistical reductionism is the main topic now under discussion. The reductionism occurs when the psychometric method is used to aggregate a set of ratings for individual "items", thereby producing a single overall rating for a complex entity such as health status or quality of life. The basic principles used for the psychometric ratings[3] are not always clearly understood by the clinicians, patients, or other people who use the ratings; and the principles may sometimes or often contradict the goals of the users. For example, the psychometric goal is to get a unidimensional measurement for an "idea" or "construct" such as intelligence, competence, political opinion, or social beliefs. This psychometric unidimensionality is contradictory to clinimetric[4] approaches that deliberately combine different attributes.

For example, consider the famous Apgar Score, created when Virginia Apgar wanted to produce a rating for the clinical condition of a newborn baby[5]. She chose five important variables: heart rate, respiratory rate, color, muscular tone, and certain reflex responses. She rated each of these a variables on a simple scale of **0, 1, 2**. She then added the five ratings to produce a score that ranges from **1** to **10**, and that is used throughout the world. I regard Apgar as the founding parent of the domain of clinimetrics; and she was very fortunate: she had no consultants to help her. If she had had the consultant guidance usually offered today, we might not have an Apgar Score. Instead, there would be an Apgar "Instrument". It would contain about 50 "items", such as "I think newborn babies are cute" (rated on a scale of **Strongly agree, ..., Strongly disagree**). "When a newborn baby turns blue, I get nervous" (rated as **Strongly agree, ..., Strongly disagree**). The instrument would have diverse statistical credentials to give accolades for "reliability" and "validity", but it would be clinically useless.

Instead, Apgar "dissected" her own clinical knowledge and judgment to produce a score that is simple, easy to use, and clinically sensible. A "sensible" score has excellent *face validity* — an attribute of paramount importance that cannot be evaluated with any known statistical procedure. Face validity is often neglected, however, when psychometric principles are used to prepare an aggregate score of weighted items. My favorite example of this problem is a sign on the outskirts of the city of Sonoma, showing the following:

Founded	1812
Elevation	560
Population	6387
Total	8759

In the psychometric quest for unidimensionality, the combination and weight of the selected items are chosen by statistical principles. According to those principles, unidimensionality is shown by the "homogeneity" of constituent items, as demonstrated by a high value of intercorrelation in a calculation called Cronbach's alpha. This calculation is unfamiliar and almost never done in clinimetric indexes, because clinicians deliberately seek to combine "heterogeneous" components, as in the *Apgar Score*, or in the categorical clusters called *TNM Stages* for the spread of cancer. The validity of those clinical ratings is not calculated statistically, but is determined from the sensibility called face validity.

Another difference in the two approaches is that psychometric principles usually prefer to avoid direct questions. In a clinimetric strategy to assess satisfaction with health care, we would ask "Do you like your doctor?" Psychometricians would ask, "Do you like doctors?" Another problem in psychometric multi-item indexes was originally noted by Nunally[6], who is one of the titans of psychometric methods. The problem is that multi-item summations can be satisfactory for denoting traits but not states. The summations are often inadequate for showing "responses" as transitions or changes in state. The inadequacy makes the multi-item indexes unsatisfactory for clinicians who want to know about the changes that follow diverse interventions, such as therapy. Clinicians usually learn about such changes by asking direct questions, such as "How are you?" of "Do you feel better or worse?". The psychometric approach, however, may fail to distinguish subtle changes because they can become obscured by the sum of multi-item components in an indirect rating scale.

Finally, in the direct clinical approach, the important components of the answers are determined by the patient, not by statistical models or by authoritative decisions. Psychometricians may then complain that the answers to these direct questions are not standardized because different patients may have different things in mind when they use such terms as *excellent* or *poor*. Nevertheless, an unstandardized answer that tells us what patients have in their mind is still better than a standardized sum, which tells us only what we academic pundits have in our mind or in our statistical models. Furthermore, when clinicians assess transitions or changes in state, a rating scale such as *much worse, ..., same, ..., much better* will be used in a reasonably standardized way to denote patients' improvement or deterioration.

My conclusion, therefore, is that although we may criticize the apparent absence of humanism in the magnificent scientific achievements of biologic reductionism, we do not restore humanism by promoting statistical reductionism and by avoiding a direct focus on the patient who is (or should be) the main concern of medical care. To determine a patients' quality of life, we can ask a professor, or a panel of "experts", or a "focus group", or the score achieved in a multi-item rating instrument for health status. The best approach, however, is to ask the patient directly. We can say, "How would you rate the way you feel about the quality of your life"; and we can record the answer on a "global" rating scale. The scale can be a mark on a visual-analog line that ranges from "could not be worse" to "could not be better". For persons who prefer the 5-categories of a "Likert-scale", the rating could be chosen from such categories as *very poor, poor, fair, good* and *excellent*.

If we want to separate the medical impact of health from the impact of all the other features of life, we can ask a second question: "How much of an effect has your state of health had on your quality of life?". This question could be answered with a choice of 5-categories that include: *Major worse effects; minor worsening; little or no effect; somewhat better*; and *major good effects*. Alternatively, the patient could put a mark on a visual analog scale that ranges from: *makes it much worse* at one end, to *makes it much better* at the other end, with *no effect* in the middle.

We could use these clinimetric methods to determine the state of a patients' quality of life and to identify changes in state. If we also want to know about diverse component entities of health and physical function, we can resort to additional approaches by asking open-ended questions, or using lists of items, including various psychometric rating scales. We can thereby take care of both sets of challenges in a suitable manner. We would have the patient rate the "whole" as a *whole*; we can then obtain individual ratings for the component parts.

We need to bear in mind, however, that most existing indexes for measuring quality of life do not measure quality of life. They measure health status. And most existing indexes for measuring health status offer an aggregate score that indicates neither the specific symptoms and distresses of a particular illness, nor the way that those specific symptoms and distresses respond to therapeutic interventions. The aggregate scores may be excellent for denoting the status of a group or population, but if individual patients are the focus of medical care, we must address those patients individually and directly to determine what their specific problems are. We can then learn what our treatments accomplish for those problems, and we can let the patients express what they want and what they have as quality of life.

REFERENCES

1. Gill, T. M., Feinstein, A.R. A critical appraisal of the quality of quality-of-life measurements. J. Amer. Med. Assn. (Aug. 24/31) 1994. 272: 619–626
2. Feinstein, A.R. Multivariable analysis. An introduction. 1996. Yale University Press. New Haven
3. Wright, J.G. and Feinstein A.R. A comparative contrast of clinimetric and psychometric methods for constructing indexes and rating scales. J. Clin. Epidemiol. (Nov.), 1992. 45: 1201–1218
4. Apgar, V. A proposal for a new method of evaluation of the newborn infant.Curr. Res. Anesth. Analg. 1953; 32: 260–267.
5. Nunally, J.C. Psychometric Theory, 2nd edn. New York: McGraw-Hill; 1978.

2

HOW DOES BASIC RESEARCH IN CANCER AND AIDS APPROACH THE CONCERN FOR QUALITY OF LIFE?

Jay A. Levy

Department of Medicine and Cancer Research Institute
University of California, School of Medicine
San Francisco, California 94143-1270

1. INTRODUCTION

Fundamental studies of cancer and AIDS are primarily directed at understanding and resolving the pathologic processes. Nevertheless, the effectiveness of the anti-cancer or anti-viral treatments developed must also consider the well-being of the patient. Measurements of quality of life, such as physical energy and mental function, need to be appreciated. For example, long-term survivors of Hodgkin's disease therapy can have substantial cognitive loss (1). Surgery for prostate cancer can lead to marked morbidity in the patient. In some cancer studies, physical well-being has been found predictive of survival, independent even of the tumor response to therapy (2). Feeling well or being in control of your health may in fact amplify the effectiveness of treatment by using the potential influence of the brain on the endocrine and immune systems and thus the pathologic process (see below).

1.1. The Approaches by Researchers

In general, basic research in cancer and AIDS can approach the concern of quality of life at six different levels (Table 1):

1. Attack the basic disease process; understand how to arrest or kill the cancer and virus-infected cells;
2. Find ways to prevent these diseases or to detect them early in development;
3. Alleviate the symptoms of cancer and AIDS that may result from products made by the affected cells or products released by an immune system responding to the malignant or virus-infected cells;

Cancer, AIDS, and Quality of Life, edited by Levy *et al.*
Plenum Press, New York, 1997

Table 1. Directions for basic research in the concern for quality

1. **Attack the basic disease processes**
2. **Find ways to prevent these diseases or to detect them early in development**
3. **Alleviate the symptoms of cancer and AIDS**
4. **Find solutions to the toxicities resulting from therapies**
5. **Stimulate the immune system against cancer and AIDS**
6. **Investigate potential processes within the brain that can enhance host responses against cancer and AIDS**

4. Find solutions to the toxicities which may occur from some of the therapies chosen for cancer and AIDS;
5. Determine the way to stimulate the immune system to fight cancer and AIDS.
6. Finally, the basic scientist can investigate biologic processes within the brain that could increase the immunologic recognition of cancer and AIDS and perhaps induce other tissues of the body to limit the pathologic processes within the host.

This latter approach appreciates the potential direct benefit of quality of life itself on controlling these diseases. It involves the current field of psychoneuroendocrinoimmunology (3), a long word embracing studies aimed at eliciting host (e.g., immune) responses that can bring clinical benefits. Certainly the overall objective of basic research is to find approaches that will eliminate or control cancer and AIDS and that will have few detrimental effects on the normal activities and well-being of the patient.

2. THE CHALLENGES OF COMBATING CANCER AND AIDS

Before considering the potential impact of research discoveries on quality of life, the overall challenge of finding solutions to cancer and AIDS should be appreciated. Basically, these two diseases, though seemingly different, share many similar properties (Table 2). For example, their pathogenesis relates to an established cellular state, either

Table 2. Similarities in the challenges of cancer and AIDS

– **Both involve an abnormal cell.**
– **Both involve recruitment of other cells into the process.**
– **Both involve modulation of antigens on the abnormal cell surface.**
– **Abnormal cell can exist in a latent state.**
– **Both are affected by apoptosis (direct or indirect).**
– **Both are affected by cytokines (direct or indirect).**
– **Cellular products can suppress host immune response.**
– **For control, both require strong cell-mediated immunity.**

transformed or virus-infected. In some cancers, moreover, a virus can be directly involved in the transformation process (e.g., Epstein-Barr virus, human T cell leukemia virus, and the human papilloma viruses). The common message is to focus therapeutic approaches on the abnormal cell, either transformed or infected.

Both cancer and AIDS can recruit other cells into the pathologic process, obviously by virus spread, or possibly by DNA transfer. With cancer, for example, observations reported over 25 years ago by Bendich and associates (4, 5) suggested that normal cells could be recruited into a tumor via the transfer of tumor cell DNA into normal cells through cytoplasmic bridges. The result is transformation of the recipient cell. While this work has been largely overlooked it perhaps merits attention, particularly with regard to polyclonal tumors.

One is reminded of the early reports of the induction of leukemia in human donor white cells during bone marrow transplants when chemotherapy and bone marrow replacement were given concurrently (6). One suggested explanation is that dying leukemic cells released DNA which was taken up by the normal donor cells leading to their transformation. The field of oncogenes was in fact discovered in part by inducing the transformation of normal cells in culture with DNA extracts from tumor cells (7) - essentially the transfer of malignant DNA to normal cells, a process resembling recruitment.

Cancer and AIDS also share the property of remaining dormant in the individual for several years (8) and then emerging, having taken advantage of either an immunocompromised host or one that has been disturbed by other lifetime factors (aging, drugs, other diseases) (9). It is recognized, for instance, that generally a physically or radiographically detectable tumor must be 1 cm^3 in size or weigh 1 gram, equal to 10^8–10^9 cells. This tumor represents 30 doublings and can take 5–7 years to develop (9). The next growth phase after its recognition consists of 10 doublings when the tumor can reach a *lethal* 1 kg mass. Thus, most of the growth cycle of a tumor is in a clinically silent state. Only during a relatively short period of time is it detected, and then only after 10 or sometimes 20 years following the initiation of the malignant cell. Early detection could, therefore, be of great benefit in cancer (see Section 4).

Similarly, with HIV infection it takes an average of 10 years for most individuals to show symptoms of infection, and for 50% to develop AIDS (10, 11). Nevertheless, the virus can be detected in some peripheral white cells and lymph nodes, although virus production is limited (12). It is the immune system, as perhaps in cancer, that maintains this latent viral state (13, 14). Understanding how the host can limit the emergence of these diseases from the silent state is obviously an important avenue of study.

Both diseases, moreover, involve processes of cell death, either necrosis or apoptosis (15). In contrast to necrosis, apoptosis, which is more common, is a normal process by which a calcium-dependent endonuclease causes selective cleavage of chromosomal DNA (15). This kind of cell death can be induced in malignant and virus-infected cells with varying types and levels of cellular products, also called cytokines. It can be caused by anti-cellular antibodies or by cytotoxic T cells attacking the cancer or virus-infected cells (16). In regard to cancer and AIDS, however, the result of apoptosis can be different. With cancer, programmed cell death, when blocked by the expression of cellular genes such as bcl-2, can create a malignant cell (17, 18). With AIDS, inhibition of apoptosis could protect a normal CD4+ cell from virus-associated indirect cell death (19). Thus, manipulation of this normal cellular process can offer directions for therapies for either disease.

Both cancer and AIDS also challenge the immune system, and in this provocation a variety of cytokines are produced by immune cells that can affect cancer cell growth (Ta-

Table 3. Cytokines and cancer

↑ Cell Growth	↓ Cell Growth
IL-4	IL-2
IL-6	Interferons
IL-10	TNF-α
TGF-β	

ble 3), and cause physical symptoms such as headaches, malaise, nausea, muscle aches, overall fatigue, and cognitive dysfunction (9, 13) (Table 4). Cancer cells and HIV-infected cells can themselves release these potentially toxic cytokines such as TNF-alpha, IL-1, or IL-6, leading to lack of appetite, gastrointestinal distress, wasting and decreased mental abilities (13, 20). Importantly, some cellular products directly suppress immune responses (13).

3. THERAPEUTIC APPROACHES TO CANCER AND AIDS

Having recognized these similarities in the biologic processes involved in cancer and AIDS, what are the therapeutic approaches (Table 5)? In cancer, attempts are made to block cell replication, destroy the transformed cell, or stop its metastases (9). Most of the current anti-cancer directions take advantage of radiation and chemical or hormonal drugs that inhibit cell division. Attempts are also being conducted to enhance the response of the immune system against these malignant cells (see Section 7). However, the arrest of cell growth or more prominently killing of the cancer cell often leads to release of products toxic to the patient and thus compromising quality of life.

An alternative approach now receiving more attention is to recognize the fact that malignant cells are usually locked in an early differentiation stage. If these cells are induced to complete their differentiation process, they may recover normal function (17). Early research in this field showed that murine chronic myelogenous leukemia cells could be induced to differentiate into normal functioning bone marrow cells and could be used to repopulate depleted bone marrow in irradiated animals (21). By inducing differentia-

Table 4. Common symptoms of cancer and AIDS

- Fever
- Malaise
- Nausea, vomiting
- Anorexia
- Fatigue
- Lethargy
- Cognitive dysfunction

Table 5. Therapeutic approaches to
cancer and AIDS

<u>**Cancer**</u>
– Surgery
– Radiation
– Chemotherapy
– Hormone therapy
– Differentiation-inducing compounds
– Immune therapy
<u>**HIV**</u>
– Antiviral - drugs, neutralizing antibodies
– Anticellular - drugs, cell-mediated immunity

tion, cancer cells may complete a regular life cycle and can then undergo normal programmed cell death. This approach has recently been highlighted by human trials with retinoic acid and phenylacetate or phenylbutyrate (22–24). Because these procedures deal with a normal cellular process, the quality of life should be much less compromised than when chemotherapy is employed.

Therapeutic approaches to HIV infection involve the drugs directed at the virus itself, particularly at its three enzymes, reverse transcriptase, integrase and protease (13). Since these enzymes are important in the replicative cycle of the virus, researchers have theorized that blocking their function would inhibit virus replication and resolve the infection. However, only a limited decrease in virus production is achieved - usually a 100-fold reduction. A major challenge of HIV and most retroviruses is their rapid growth and their mutation potential (13). Any viruses replicating in the face of therapy can undergo many mutations (e.g., 10 per replication cycle), and emerge as drug-resistant virus strains (13, 25), or viruses that "home out" and cause disease in certain tissues such as the brain and bowel (13). Most importantly, the current drugs block only *de novo* infection by the virus, but the chronically-infected cells, containing the integrated viral genome, continue to divide and release virus particles - up to 1000 per day (26). These cells should be the major target of therapy (27) as are cancer cells. Thus, while short-term benefits (measured in months) may be achieved with the anti-HIV drugs currently used, their effect may not lead to a greatly enhanced survival.

In some cases of HIV infection, antiretroviral drugs such as zidovudine (or AZT) have improved quality of life (281, 29, 30). Appetite returns, weight gain occurs, and in some patients, signs of AIDS dementia are reversed (31). But, the toxic side effects of these drugs is usually problematic (32, 33). In fact, when quality of life enters the evaluation of a clinical trial, the efficacy of AZT in patients with AIDS and AIDS related complex can be greatly reduced. In some clinical trials, no significant differences were observed between treated and untreated groups after a year of therapy (29). Furthermore, in a study of asymptomatic individuals receiving daily 500 mg of zidovudine, a marked reduction in quality of life was observed due to the side effects of therapy particularly toxicity to the bone marrow (34). Thus, any positive effects of therapy were compromised by the reduction in quality of life. Such harmful effects need to be countered either by decreasing the drug dosage, using multiple drugs at low toxicity or finding approaches to avoid the toxicities. Most importantly, a variety of anti-HIV therapies need to be developed especially those directed at controlling the infected cell (27).

4. EARLY DETECTION OF CANCER AND AIDS

In a related topic (alluded to in Section 2), research efforts are continually being directed at finding ways of detecting cancer or HIV early so that appropriate drugs or surgery can be given before there is a large tumor or viral load. For example, the test for prostate-specific antigen (or PSA) alerts physicians to the possibility of prostatic cancer (35–37). That test has now led to a markedly increased number of prostate operations in the United States. Whether these operations are necessary is an important question. The procedure has caused great morbidity, including incontinence and impotence in many subjects undergoing the surgery. Clinicians are now debating the true benefits of the PSA test (38, 39). If strongly positive, it appears to reflect the extrusion already of the cancer cell through the blood vessel wall. Thus, metastases have most likely occurred. Many urologists, therefore, now recommend that only individuals under 65 with a high PSA have surgery, since in older patients this cancer can remain dormant for 20–30 years without evidence of metastases or clinical symptoms. Up to 30% of men over the age of 60 at autopsy have occult prostatic cancer (40).

Similarly, detection of tumors of the breast involves routine procedures such as mammograms which can lead to widespread surgery in this common cancer of women. Initially, radical mastectomy was undertaken. Now fortunately clinical and basic research studies have shown that lumpectomy statistically gives similar results (41, 42) without the disfigurement associated with the former operation. The recent possibility of genetic screening for the breast cancer gene (43) raises new issues about the best response to a positive result. Radical mastectomy, which some women may choose, could be ineffective since this operation cannot remove all mammary cells. Thus, when and what approaches to choose in breast cancer are major unresolved questions.

Researchers need to appreciate the stages involved in the evolution of cancer (Figure 1). The cell can begin from an *in situ* lesion that can remain latent for years (and sometimes a lifetime), and then proceed through a stepwise pattern to emerge as a malignancy. Such observations have been made with cervical and anal cancers caused by the human papilloma virus (44) and with bowel malignancies, associated with concurrent expression of different oncogenes (45). Breast cancer often progresses from hormone dependence to independence (46). Thus, understanding the biology of the cancer cell and what type of small lesions are more likely to have a malignant and metastatic phenotype can influence the extent of surgery and therapy recommended and bring great clinical benefits. Until then, attention should be given to warnings about conducting and over-interpreting such early detection methods.

With HIV, early detection can be realized through analyses of viral RNA and infected cells in the blood (13), but drugs are not yet available that can curtail this infection

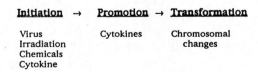

Figure 1. Steps involved in tumor development. A variety of stimuli can initiate the malignant process. For emergence into a transformed cell, promotion of this precancerous cell must occur and is often effected by increased cytokine-induced cell proliferation. The resultant enhanced cell division will permit chromosomal changes that lead to autonomous out-growth of a malignant cell.

before as many as 250 billion white cells in the body are infected, particularly in lymphoid tissue (12). The estimated time for such viral spread is 7–14 days after initial transmission. Thus, therapeutic approaches should be aimed at the earliest period after infection in hopes of limiting virus spread - stopping not only the new infection by HIV, but most importantly virus production by the already infected cell (27).

5. RESEARCH APPROACHES TO COUNTER THE TOXIC EFFECTS OF CELLULAR PRODUCTS ASSOCIATED WITH CANCER AND AIDS (TABLE 6)

Finding methods to limit the toxicity of cytokines or other cellular products released by cancer and HIV-infected cells or by immune cells responding to these diseases (Table 3) has received recent attention. As examples, recent clinical trials with pentoxifylline, the anti-TNF-α drug (47) may be beneficial in blocking some of the side effects of TNF-α (48), such as wasting and cell toxicity, which for some investigators is the major cause of AIDS symptomatology (20). Most recently, the controversial drug, thalidomide, has offered some promise in countering the harmful side effects of TNF-α (49). Other attempts at such immune modulation include the use of antibodies against specific cytokines (50).

6. APPROACHES TO COUNTER THE TOXICITIES OF TREATMENT (TABLE 6)

Among the most common feared side effects of treatment for cancer and AIDS are nausea and vomiting. Research into anti-emetics has brought forth a variety of products, particularly 5-HT$_3$ receptor antagonists, which can greatly reduce these symptoms in cancer patients receiving toxic therapies (51). The drugs can decrease the discomforts of chemotherapy and permit adequate food and nutrient supplementation.

To counter the toxic effects of drugs on the bone marrow, G-CSF, GM-CSF, erythropoietin, and recently thrombopoietin produced through genetic engineering procedures can be helpful (52–54). G-CSF and GM-CSF have led to a reduction in the risk of hospitalization for febrile neutropenia. Erythropoietin reduces the need for transfusions and decreases infections resulting from a poor functioning immune system. Thrombopoietin can help with platelet losses.

Table 6. Approaches to symptoms of cancer and AIDS and side effects of therapy

- **Anti-emetics**
- **Anti-cytokines**
- **Growth factor replacement**
- **Bone marrow replacement**
- **Gene therapy - p-glycoprotein**
- **Immune modulation**

In some cases, myeloid growth factors have helped engraftment with allogeneic bone marrow transplantation. In fact, bone marrow transplantation is now being considered not only for leukemias (55), but as you know, for the replacement of hematopoietic cells lost during chemotherapy. In some trials, normal bone marrow stem cells are receiving constructs carrying the p-glycoprotein that induces resistance to chemotherapeutic drugs (56, 57). Given to the patient, higher doses of anti-cancer drugs can be tolerated since the normal cells are protected from drug toxicity. The most recent innovative trial of a baboon bone marrow in an AIDS patient (58) illustrates the new approaches being studied for these diseases. Perhaps the discovery of the facilitator cell (a new immune cell in the T cell series that helps engraftment) (59) will widen the use of bone marrow transplants in cancer and AIDS.

The interplay of cellular components of the immune system and their products offer other approaches to counter toxic effects of therapy as well as to control the diseases directly. All these research advances aimed at modifying the pathologic effects of cancer and HIV infected cells and the toxicities of treatment, attempt to reconstitute the natural antitumor or antiviral resources in the body that have been compromised.

7. APPROACHES TO INCREASE THE IMMUNE RESPONSE TO CANCER AND AIDS

A major strategy for controlling cancer and AIDS should be to increase the host's immune response against these diseases. This direction, because it uses a natural system, should have fewer deleterious effects on a patient's quality of life. Cellular immune responses, reflected by CD8+ cells, macrophages (and other antigen-presenting cells) and NK cells, have the best potential in immunotherapy because they attack the cancer cell and the virus-infected cell.

In cancer, IL-2 and GM-CSF delivered with vaccines and certain therapies have offered hope in enhancing cell-mediated responses against the tumor cells (60, 61). Replacement therapy with LAK or TIL cells (primarily CD8+ T cells) directed against specific cancer cells is also being actively explored (62).

In HIV, we have observed that CD8+ cells from HIV-infected individuals living for more than ten years (for some,18 years) can control virus replication in the infected cell by production of a novel CD8+ cell antiviral factor (CAF) (13, 14, 63). This cellular product blocks HIV transcription (64). Work in our laboratory has demonstrated that IL-2, a CD4+ cell cytokine, can increase this CD8+ cell anti-HIV response (65). These observations offer approaches for future therapy for HIV infection either through direct cytokine treatment , such as IL-2 (66) or CAF or the induction and maintenance of CAF production by host CD8+ cells.

One other cytokine that enhances cell mediated immunity is IL12 (67, 68) and it has been recently evaluated in Phase 1 clinical trials. The early results were disappointing since ill effects were observed in humans (69) mostly due to the induction by IL-12 of TNF-α (70). Lower doses of IL-12 are now being evaluated. Thus, dramatically, it was observed that going from the workbench to clinical trials requires not only careful planning of protocols, but also the recognition of the potential consequences the laboratory finding can have on the patient.

Most importantly, through basic research, the network of immune responses that reflects an interaction of many cytokines and cellular components is being better defined (13). The eventual hope is that deficits in certain areas can be relieved through future discoveries from basic research. The ultimate objective is to find a means of inducing the appropriate immune response of the affected individual against the cancer or HIV-infected cells. Presumedly, by harnessing such a natural process, fewer toxicities will be encountered and quality of life will be maintained.

8. THE NEURO-ENDOCRINE-IMMUNE SYSTEM INTERACTIONS

One important facet to consider in the approaches used against cancer and AIDS is the potential influence of the central nervous system or the mind on the immune and endocrine systems (3, 71). While sometimes given less attention or even derided, the possibility that thought processes could affect disease progression should not be underestimated. Stress, for example, can cause many symptoms in people (72), including outbreaks of herpesvirus infections. The role of a depressed immune system during stress has been recognized (71, 73–75).

The potential influence of the mind on the body has been suggested for centuries (76) - as far back as Ayurveda in India (77). Over 100 years ago, Daniel Tuke in his treatise, *Illustrations on the Influence of the Mind on the Body in Health and Disease*, emphasized the effects of the brain on the vasculative and muscles (78). Only recently in this century have new insights into the now recognized brain-endocrine-immune system axis been obtained from basic research. It must be appreciated that the immune system is not an autonomous entity but continually sends signals and responds to messages from the central nervous system as well as endocrine tissues. The terms neuropeptides, hormones and lymphokines suggest that they are unique to their respective tissue, but we now know that many of these substances can be made in diverse tissues.

To expect such an intercommunication among these three systems, some physical or chemical connections should be found. Toward this objective, experimental studies and immuno-electron microscopy have demonstrated nerve fibers that enervate all lymphoid organs throughout the body. They can be detected adjacent to lymphocytes, macrophages and smooth muscle cells of arterioles (79). These nerve endings contain a variety of neuropeptides that in many cases share homologies with cytokines released by immune cells and hormones produced by endocrine organs (3, 79). For example, interferon, ACTH and endorphins have structural similarities. The list of factors shared by the nervous, en-

Table 7. Production of neuropeptides, hormones, and cytokines by the nervous, endocrine, and immune systems

	Neural	Endocrine	Immune
Interleukin-1	Astrocytes	-	Macrophage
Somatostatin	Frontal cortex	Pancreas	Basophil
Substance P	Spinal cord	Pituitary	-
Vasoactive intestinal peptide (VIP)	Hypothalamus	Ovary, testes	Neutrophil
ACTH	-	Pituitary	Lymphocyte
Endorphin, Enkephalin	+	-	Lymphocyte

Summarized from O'Dorisio, M., Chapter 14, The Neuroendocrine-Immune Network, 1990, CRC Press, Inc.

docrine and immune systems keeps growing (Table 7). The inference is that these cellular products help form the basis of communication among these three organ systems.

Another major discovery linking the nervous, endocrine and immune systems was the recognition in the early 1970's of receptors on lymphocytes for a variety of neuropeptides, such as endorphins (80, 81) (Table 8). Since then receptors for many hormones as well as neurotransmitters have been identified on several immune cells (Table 9) and on cells from the endocrine and nervous systems (82). The neurotransmitters and their cellular targets support suggestions of such intercommunications from psychological studies. For example, passive versus active coping has correlated with breast tumor growth and metastasis and a greater incidence of cervical neoplasms in women (83).

The interactions among these three systems provide further evidence that thought processes are biochemical, and that psycho-social and environmental stimuli can influence neuropeptide production and thereby immune function. Thus, three important prerequisites for a direct effect of the brain on the immune system have been found: 1) peripheral nerve enervation of lymphoid tissues, 2) the presence in the nerve fibers of neuropeptides, and 3) receptors for these neuropeptides on immune cells.

One example of how enervated nerve fibers and their neuropeptides might be responsible for symptoms is psychogenic arthritis. The nerve fibers localized in the joints contain a high concentrations of substance P (84). Substance P creates inflammatory changes when injected into the joint cavity. Under certain psychological conditions, a high release of substance P from these nerve fibers could conceivably induce development of an arthritis-like condition, for example, juvenile pseudo-rheumatoid arthritis.

A similar type of connection has been elucidated between the brain and gastrointestinal system (85). Much evidence now suggests that a separate functioning enteric nervous system (ENS) can be defined that can regulate function in the bowel even in the absence of the brain. The immune components of the bowel would be under similar communications with nerve endings from the ENS.

The relationship between the nervous system and the lymphoid system is well-illustrated in the developing embryo (86). Mesenchymal cells derived from the neural crest (the site for nervous system development) contribute the epithelial components in the thymus within which thymocytes originating in fetal liver or bone marrow develop. In the absence of the neural crest no thymus is formed and the immune system is markedly limited in its development. A reflection of this interaction is the finding of the Thy-1 and CD4 antigen on T lymphocytes and cells of the brain in rodents (87), and humans respectively (88). Moreover, as noted above, cytokines released by lymphocytes are also found produced by counterparts in the brain such as astrocytes and oligodendrocytes (13, 88).

Table 8. Neuropeptide receptors on immune cells[*]

Adregenic - α,β	Seratonin
Cholinergic (acetylcholine)	Somatostatin
Dopamine	Substance P
Endorphins, enkephalins	Vasopresin
Melatonin	VIP
Neurotensin	

[*]T and B lymphocytes, monocytes/macrophages; NK cells and/or neutrophils.

Table 9. Hormone receptors on lymphocytes

ACTH	Progestin
Corticosteroids	Prolactin
Estrogen	Testosterone
Growth hormone	Thyroxin
Insulin	TSH
Melatonin	
Oxytocin	

A functional thymus is essential as well for the normal hypothalamic- pituitary axis. For example, athymic nude mice have both the T cell defects noted above, and also depressed levels of thyroxin and gonadatropin (89). Return of thymus tissue to the animals restores both immune and endocrine functions.

Other studies have indicated how both neural and hormonal factors can influence immunologic responses to cancer and infectious organisms (Table 10). In some cases, they can enhance lymphocyte proliferation and in others they limit this response (3, 71, 75). The endogenous morphine-like substances, endorphins and enkephalins, for example, can both increase and decrease the immune response depending on their concentration and the cell type involved (3, 90). The pineal neurohormone, melatonin, can counter the immune suppressing effects of stress by inducing CD4+ cells to release opiate-like substances (91). These same natural substances produced locally can reduce the pain and discomfort of cancer and AIDS patients.

For its part, the immune system via cytokine release can influence the brain through the hypothalamus to secrete various substances in response to an immune signal. IL-1, for example, can stimulate the pituitary-adrenal axis to influence the release of glycocorticosteroids. These same adrenal hormones can at high level reduce IL-1 production. Some cytokines may directly cause the fatigue observed in cancer and AIDS patients. The site of

Table 10. Immune functions affected by neuropeptides

B cell
- **Antibody production**
- **Cytokine production**

T cell
- **Proliferation**
- **Cytotoxic activity**
- **Cytokine production**

NK cell
- **Cell killing (cancer or virus-infected)**
- **ADCC**

Macrophages
- **Phagocytosis**
- **Chemotaxis**
- **ADCC**

ADCC: antibody-dependent cellular cytotoxicity

fatigue is in the hypothalamus and is associated in some studies with high plasma levels of IL-1 and TNFα. IL-1 (produced by macrophages), interferon, and TNF-α have been shown to affect sleep wave patterns (71, 92, 93).

Conceivably, products of the immune system influence the brain's control of nerve endings. It has been observed, for instance, that the release of noradrenaline from nerve fibers in the spleen is decreased during infection (94). This reduction in neuropeptide production, most likely induced by products of the immune system, leads to an enhanced and beneficial immune response.

In this regard, stress, frequently cited as a cause of immune suppression, has been found associated with not only steroid hormone release, but also production of several neuropeptides. They could be responsible for the decreased cellular proliferation and reduced macrophage and NK tumoricidal activity reported during times of stress, bereavement, and depression (73–75, 95). Most recently, acute stress, formerly believed to decrease immunity, as reflected by reduced peripheral blood lymphocyte and NK cell numbers (73), has been found to increase lymphocyte proliferation and immune responses. It is chronic stress that is associated with a compromised immune system reflected by decreased resistance to tumors or infectious organisms.

Some investigators summarize the major function of the immune system as a sensory organ (96, 97) (Figure 2). It has the receptors for recognizing non-cognitive stimuli (e.g., infectious organisms) that would not be recognized by the brain. This information on infection is forwarded by the immune system to the neuroendocrine system by cytokines or hormones released by the immune cells (97). Subsequent changes in physiological as well as immunologic status takes place. Thus, on one hand, psychological or mental stress would be the cognitive stimuli that direct responses from the CNS to affect endocrine and immune function. Release of corticosteroids, for example, can affect immune function (75). On the other hand, invading organisms or toxins would be the stimuli to the immune system via cytokines to alert the CNS and bring about neurologic as well as endocrine responses.

Moreover, notably, without CNS involvement, the immune and endocrine systems can still interact. Studies have shown that viral infection of an animal that has no pituitary gland still induces steroid production that affects the immune response (89, 98). It is assumed that the virus induces in lymphocytes the release of an ACTH-like substance which can affect cortisone production by adrenal glands directly if this response is not elicited indirectly by the brain. Some data also suggest that thyrotropin-releasing hormone can also be produced by immune cells and lead directly to thyroid hormone production (89).

Results with conditioning experiments underline these sensory functions of both the neurologic and immune systems. Based on the earlier observations of Metal'nikov and Chorine (99), Ader and Cohen (75, 100–102) showed the effect of a conditioning stimulus (one that the subject can feel) and an unconditioning stimulus (one that is not felt) on immune responses in rodents. One study in cancer involved giving the odor of camphor as the conditioned stimulus together with poly IC as the unconditioned stimulus. This latter compound induces interferon production that increases NK cell killing of tumor cells (103). In this experiment, when the tumor cells were injected along with the smell of camphor alone, only those animals previously given the smell of camphor and poly IC once a day for 9 days showed prominent NK cell anti-cancer activity and longer survival (103).

In other conditioning experiments designed to avoid the possible role of stress from a noxious odor, the sweet taste of saccharine replaced camphor; similar results were

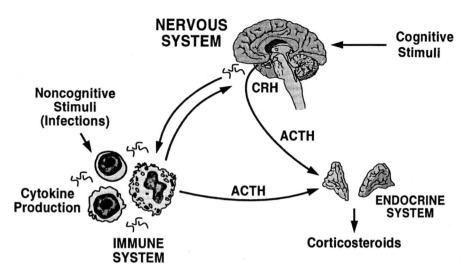

Figure 2. Interactions of the nervous, endocrine and immune systems. Cognitive or non-cognitive stimuli can directly affect the nervous system or the immune system, respectively, and lead to processes that induce responses in the endocrine system. Shown here, for example, is the ability of the stimuli to induce ACTH production by either the brain or the immune system with subsequent induction of corticosteroid production by the endocrine system (adapted from Blalock, 1985).

found (104). A well-known study was conducted with a young female patient suffering from systemic lupus erythematosus (105). This young girl received cod liver oil as the conditioning stimulus (taste) concomitant with the drug cyclophosphamide used to reduce T cell hyperreactivity. Following receipt of this regimen for several months, the girl was given only cod liver oil and a similar reduction in hyperactive T cells was shown. The ultimate result was a decrease in the amount of the toxic drug cyclophosphamide needed to bring clinical benefit to the patient. Although only one clinical case study has been reported, this approach merits further attention to finding treatments that benefit quality of life.

One other important point about this nervous-endocrine-immune system interaction should be appreciated. If we accept that positive signals from the brain can help the immune and endocrine systems respond to cancer and AIDS, then negative signals may have the opposite effects. Just as there may be abnormalities in certain organ systems developed in the host over time, abnormal responses in the brain might induce the immune or endocrine dysfunctions that lead to cancer development (e.g., hormone-dependent tumors). Whether we can reverse the negative signals from the brain as we have attempted to do with the endocrine and immune systems is a further challenge to basic research.

While still in its infancy, the potential of mental or neurologic interaction with the endocrine and immune systems leading to immunologic control of diseases is becoming apparent (106). Basic research may eventually be able to explain some of the miraculous healings that have been documented with cancer (107). Furthermore, these approaches once developed would utilize natural responses of the body and thus should have minimal effects on quality of life.

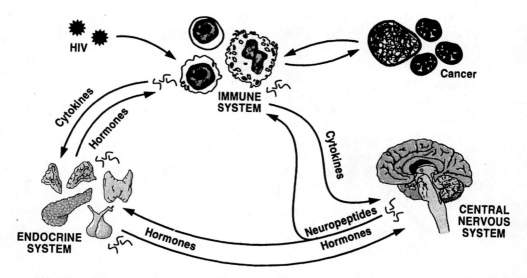

Figure 3. The multi-potential cell. The hypothesis is presented that cells may be inducible under certain conditions to express a variety of cellular products that are generally recognized as secretions from other tissues and organ systems.

9. CONCLUSIONS

Basic science must continue to look at the major pathways involved in cancer and AIDS and find solutions for arresting these pathologic processes. This work will lead to effective approaches to resolve the side effects of cancer and AIDS - such as fatigue, nausea, vomiting, GI distress and cognitive dysfunction. Throughout all these efforts, scientists must appreciate as well the advantages of promoting good quality of life - essentially

The Multi-Purpose Cell

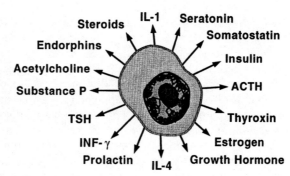

Figure 4. The neuro-endocrine-immune system axis. Viral diseases such as HIV and cancer challenge the immune system leading to the production of cellular products or cytokines that can affect both the endocrine system and the central nervous system. The central nervous system will produce neuropeptides as well as hormones that can have an effect on the immune system or on the endocrine system. Likewise, the endocrine system can produce hormones that will act on the immune system and the central nervous system. Through this intercommunication among these various tissues, appropriate responses to stress, infectious organisms, and other stimuli can be achieved.

recalling the Latin expression, *mens sana, in corpore sano*, "a sound mind in a sound body." Effective direct therapy against cancer and AIDS with the maintenance of personal comfort can provide the additional potential of a healthy mind continually helping to combat the pathologic processes involved. Beneficial interactions of the central nervous system with the endocrine and immune systems could assure the normal functioning of the many organs in the body.

One could even imagine in the future harnessing the full potential of any cell in the body to perform many functions if required. As you are aware, neuropeptides released by the brain can be produced by the immune system. The immune system releases cytokines that are also produced in the brain. Insulin is made by the pancreas and is also released by lymphocytes. Perhaps a wide vista of novel approaches can be developed through basic research in the years ahead by which other cells of the body can be induced to take on the challenge of cells that have lost this specialized function (Figure 3). Lymphocytes or lung cells might provide necessary hormones or cytokines for attacking the malignant undifferentiated cancer cells or cells infected by an invading virus.

Long-term survivors of cancer and HIV infection have been able to mount a controlling response to their diseases and maintain a clinically healthy state. The mystery of their ability to ward off disease or keep it under control (sometimes for 15–20 years) is a major area for continued basic research. It involves approaches that envelop the issues of quality of life. Such research, which considers fundamental studies in biology and biochemistry certainly must also appreciate the psycho-neuro-endocrino-immunology axis that functions to assure a healthy state (Figure 4). Together, the new findings could bring the most promising results in conquering these two devastating diseases in the 21st century.

ACKNOWLEDGMENTS

I would like to thank Drs. Ellen Koenig, Stuart Levy, Rodger Winn, and Edward Goetzl for their helpful comments on this paper. Leslie Compere helped with the graphics. Christine Beglinger is thanked for her assistance in the preparation of the manuscript.

REFERENCES

1. Devlen J, Maquire P, Phillips P. Psychological problems associated with diagnosis and treatment of lymphomas. I. Retrospective study. British Medical Journal 1987;295:953–954.
2. Coates A, Gebski V, Signorini D, Murray P, McNeil D, Byrne M. Prognostic value of quality of life scores during chemotherapy for advanced breast cancer. Journal of Clinical Oncology 1992;10:1833–1828.
3. Ader R, Felton DL, Cohen N. Psychoneuroimmunology.San Diego: Academic Press, Inc., 1991
4. Bendich A, Borenfreund E, Honda Y, Steinglass M. Cell transformation and the genesis of cancer. Archives of Environmental Health 1969;19:157–166.
5. Bendich A, Vizoso AD, Harris RG. Intercellular bridges between mammalian cells in culture. Proceedings of the National Academy of Sciences (USA) 1967;57:1029–1035.
6. Thomas ED, Storb R, Clift RA, et al. Bone-marrow transplantation. New England Journal of Medicine 1975;292:895–902.
7. Rasheed S. Retroviruses and oncogenes. In: Levy JA, ed. The Retroviridae. New York: Plenum Press, 1995;4:293–408.
8. Yefenof E, Picker LJ, Scheuermann RH, Tucker TF, Vitetta ES, Uhr JW. Cancer dormancy: isolation and characterization of dormant lymphoma cells. Proceedings of the National Academy of Sciences (USA) 1993;90:1829–1833.
9. DeVita T, Jr., Hellman S, Rosenberg SA, ed. Cancer, Principles and Practic of Oncology. 4th ed. Philadelphia: Lippincott, 1993:

10. Rutherford GW, Lifson AR, Hessol NA. Course of HIV-1 infection in a cohort of homosexual and bisexual men: an 11 year follow up study. British Medical Journal 1990;301:1183–1188.

11. Buchbinder SP, Katz MH, Hessol NA, O'Malley PM, Holmberg SD. Long-term HIV-1 infection without immunologic progression. AIDS 1994;8:1123–1128.

12. Embretson J, Zupancic M, Ribas JL, et al. Massive covert infection of helper T lymphocytes and macrophages by HIV during the incubation period of AIDS. Nature 1993;362:359–362.

13. Levy JA. HIV and the Pathogenesis of AIDS.Washington, DC: American Society of Microbiology, 1994

14. Levy JA. HIV pathogenesis and long-term survival. AIDS 1993;7:1401–1410.

15. Tomei LD, Cope FO. Apoptosis: The molecular Basis of Cell Death.Cold Spring Harbor: Cold Spring Harbor Laboratory Press, 1991

16. Berke G. Unlocking the secrets of CTL and NK cells. Immunology Today 1995;16:343–346.

17. Sawyers CL, Denny CT, Witte ON. Leukemia and the disruption of normal hematopoiesis. Cell 1991;64:337–350.

18. Nunez G, Seto M, Seremetis S, et al. Growth- and tumor-promoting effects of deregulated BCL2 in human B-lymphoblastoid cells. Proceedings of the National Academy of Sciences (USA) 1989;86:4589–4593.

19. Ameisen JC. Programmed cell death (apoptosis) and cell survival regulation: relevance to AIDS and cancer. AIDS 1994;8:1197–1213.

20. Matsuyama T, Kobayashi N, Yamamoto N. Cytokines and HIV infection: Is AIDS a tumor necrosis factor disease? AIDS 1991;5:1405–1417.

21. Sachs L. Control of normal cell differentiation and the phenotypic reversion of malignancy in myeloid leukaemia. Nature 1978;274:535–539.

22. Degos L, Dombret H, Chomienna C, et al. All-*trans*-retinoic acid as a differentiating agent in the treatment of acute promyelocytic leukemia. Blood 1995;85:2643–2653.

23. Dmitrovsky E, Markman M, Marks PA. Clinical use of differentiating agents in cancer therapy. Cancer Chemotherapy and Biological Response Modifiers 1990;11:303–320.

24. Huang ME, Ye YC, Chen SR, et al. Use of all-trans retinoic acid in the treatment of acute promyelocytic leukemia. Blood 1988;72:567–572.

25. Richman DD. HIV drug resistance. AIDS Research and Human Retroviruses 1992;8:1065–1071.

26. Levy JA, Ramachandran B, Barker E, Guthrie J, Elbeik T. Plasma viral load, CD4+ cell counts, and HIV-1 production by cells. Science 1996;271:670–671.

27. Levy JA. HIV research: a need to focus on the right target. Lancet 1995;345:1619–1621.

28. Volberding PA, Lagakos SW, Koch MA, et al. Zidovudine in asymptomatic human immunodeficiency virus infection: A controlled trial in persons with fewer than 500 CD4-positive cells per cubic millimeter. New England Journal of Medicine 1990;322:941–949.

29. Wu AW, Mathews WC, Brysk LT, et al. Quality of life in a placebo-controlled trial of zidovudine in patients with AIDS and AIDS-related complex. Journal of Acquired Immune Deficiency Syndromes 1990;3:683–690.

30. Fischl MA, Richman DD, Grieco MH, et al. The efficacy of azidothymidine (AZT) in the treatment of patients with AIDS and AIDS-related complex. A double blind placebo controlled trial. New England Journal of Medicine 1987;317:185–191.

31. Portegies P. AIDS dementia complex: a review. Journal of Acquired Immune Deficiency Syndromes 1994;7:S38-S49.

32. Gelber RD, Lenderking WR, Cotton DJ, et al. Quality of life evaluation in a clinical trial of zidovudine therapy in patients with mildly symptomatic HIV infection. Annals of Internal Medicine 1992;116:961–966.

33. Richman DD, Fischl MA, Grieco MH, et al. The toxicity of azidothymidine (AZT) in the treatment of patients with AIDS and AIDS-related complex. New England Journal of Medicine 1987;317:192–197.

34. Lenderking WR, Gelber RD, Cotton DJ, et al. Evaluation of the quality of life associated with zidovudine treatment in asymptomatic human immunodeficiency virus infection. New England Journal of Medicine 1994;330:738–743.

35. Catalona WJ, Smith DS, Ratliff TL. Measurement of prostate-specific antigen in serum as a screening test for prostate cancer. New England Journal of Medicine 1991;324:1156.

36. Catalona WJ, Smith DS, Ratliff TL. Detection of organ-confined prostate cancer is increased through prostate specific antigen based screening. Journal of the American Medical Association 1993;270:948.

37. Thompson IM, Optenberg SA. An overview cost-utility analysis of prostate cancer screening. Oncology 1995;9:141–145.

38. Kramer BS, Brown ML, Prorok PC, Potosky AL, Gohagan JK. Prostate cancer screening: what we know and what we need to know. annals of Internal Medicine 1993;119:914–923.

39. Krahn MD, Mahoney JE, Eckman MH, Trachtenberg J, Pauker SG, Detsky AS. Screening for prostate cancer. Journal of the american Medical Association 1994;272:773–780.
40. Franks LM. Latent carcinoma of the prostate. Journal of Pathology and Bacteriology 1954;68:603.
41. Fisher B, Anderson S, Redmond CK, Wolmark N, Wickerham DL, Cronin WM. Reanalysis and results after 12 years of follow-up in a randomized clinical trial comparing total mastectomy with lumpectomy with or without irradiation in the treatment of breast cancer. New England Journal of Medicine 1995;333:1456–1461.
42. Veronesi U, Banfi A, Salvadori B, et al. Breast conservation is the treatment of choice in small breast cancer: long-term results of a randomized trial. European Journal of Cancer 1990;26:668–670.
43. Collins FS. BRCA1 - lots of mutations, lots of dilemmas. New England Journal of Medicine 1996;334:186–188.
44. zur Hausen H. Human papillomaviruses in the pathogenesis of anogenital cancer. Virology 1991;184:9–13.
45. Vogelstein B, Kinzler KW. The multistep nature of cancer. Trends in Genetics 1993;9:138–141.
46. Murphy LC. Antiestrogen action and growth factor regulation. Breast Cancer Research and Treatment 1994;31:61–71.
47. Ward A, Clissold SP. Pentoxifylline: a review of its pharmacodynamic and pharmacokinetic properties, and its therapeutic efficacy. Drugs 1987;34:50–97.
48. Dezube BJ, Lederman MM, Spritzler JG, et al. High-dose pentoxifylline in patients with AIDS: inhibition of tumor necrosis factor production. Journal of Infectious Diseases 1995;171:1628–1632.
49. Sampaio EP, Sarno EN, Galilly R, Cohn ZA, Kaplan G. Thalidomide selectively inhibits tumor necrosis factor-alpha production by stimulated human monocytes. Journal of Experimental Medicine 1991;173:699–703.
50. Clerici M, Wynn TA, Berzofsky JA, et al. Role of interleukin-10 in T helper cell dysfunction in asymptomatic individuals infected with the human immunodeficiency virus. Journal of Clinical Investigation 1994;93:768–775.
51. Grunberg SM. Economic impact of antiemesis. Oncology 1995;9:155–160.
52. Lyman GH, Balducci L. A cost analysis of hematopoietic colony-stimulating factors. Oncology 1995;9:85–91.
53. Glaspy JA. Economic outcomes associated with the use of hematopoietic growth factors. Oncology 1995;9:93–105.
54. Henry DH, Beall GN, Benson CA, et al. Recombinant human erythropoietin in the treatment of anemia associated with human immunodeficiency virus (HIV) infection and zidovudine therapy. Annals of Internal Medicine 1992;117:739–748.
55. Winer EP, Sutton LM. Quality of life after bone marrow transplantation. Oncology 1994;8:19–27.
56. Ling V. P-glycoprotein and resistance to anticancer drugs. Cancer 1992;69:2603–2609.
57. Sorrentino BP, Brandt SJ, Bodine D, et al. Selection of drug-resistant bone marrow cells *in vivo* after retroviral transfer of human MDRI. Science 1992;257:99–102.
58. Altman LK. Hospital to release patient who received baboon cells; man survives riskiest stage of experiment. The New York Times 1996 January 4, 1996:C19.
59. Kaufman CL, Gaines BA, Ildstad ST. Xenotransplantation. Annual Review of Immunology 1995;13:339–367.
60. Schmidt W, Schweighoffer T, herbst E, et al. Cancer vaccines: the interleukin 2 dosage effect. Proceedings of the National Academy of Sciences (USA) 1995;92:4711–4714.
61. Bernstein ZP, Porter MM, Gould M, et al. Prolonged administration of low-dose interleukin-2 in human immunodeficiency virus-associated malignancy results in selective expansion of innate immune effectors without significant clinical toxicity. Blood 1995;86:3287–3294.
62. Rosenberg SA, Packard BS, Aebersold PM. Use of tumor-infiltrating lymphocytes and interleukin-2 in the immunotherapy of patients with metastic melanoma: a preliminary report. New England Journal of Medicine 1988;319:1676–1680.
63. Mackewicz C, Levy JA. CD8+ cell anti-HIV activity: Nonlytic suppression of virus replication. AIDS Research and Human Retroviruses 1992;8:1039–1050.
64. Mackewicz CE, Blackbourn DJ, Levy JA. CD8+ cells suppress HIV replication by inhibiting viral transcription. Proceedings of the National Academy of Sciences (USA) 1995;92:2308–2312.
65. Barker E, Mackewicz CE, Levy JA. Effects of TH1 and TH2 cytokines on CD8+ cell response against human immunodeficiency virus: implications for long-term survival. Proceedings of the National Academy of Sciences (USA) 1995;92:11135–11139.
66. Kovacs JA, Baseler M, Dewar RJ, et al. Increases in CD4 T lymphocytes with intermittent courses of interleukin-2 in patients with human immunodeficiency virus infection. New England Journal of Medicine 1995;332:567–575.

67. Clerici M, Lucey DR, Berzofsky JA, et al. Restoration of HIV-specific cell-mediated immune responses by interleukin-12 in vitro. Science 1993;262:1721–1724.

68. Scott P. IL-12: initiation cytokine for cell-mediated immunity. Science 1993;260:496–497.

69. Hall SS. IL-12 at the crossroads. Science 1995;268:1432–1434.

70. Orange JS, Salazar-Mather TP, Opal SM, et al. Mechanism of interleukin 12-mediated toxicities during experimental viral infections: role of tumor necrosis factor and glucocorticoids. Journal of Experimental Medicine 1995;181:901–914.

71. Solomon GF. Psychoneuroimmunology: interactions between central nervous system and immune system. Journal of Neuroscience Research 1987;18:1–9.

72. Seyle H. The Stress of Life.Toronto: McGraw-Hill Book Co., 1956

73. Evans DL, Folds JD, Petitto JM, et al. Circulating natural killer cell phenotypes in men and women with major depression. Archives of General Psychiatry 1992;49:388–395.

74. Stein M, Miller AH, Trestman RL. Depression and the Immune System. In: Ader R, Felten DL, Cohen N, ed. Psychoneuroimmunology. San Diego: Academic Press, Inc., 1991: 897–930.

75. Cohen S, Williamson GM. Stress and infectious disease in humans. Psychological Bulletin 1991;109:5–24.

76. Lucretius. On the Nature of the Universe. New York: Penguin Books, 1951 (Latham RF, ed.)

77. Chopra D. Quantum Healing.New York: Bantam Books, 1989

78. Tuke DT. Illustrations of the Influence of the Mind Upon the Body.London: Churchill, 1884

79. Felten SY, Felten DL. Innervation of lymphoid tissue. In: Ader R, Felten DL, Cohen N, ed. Psychoneuroimmunology. San Diego: Academic Press, Inc., 1991: 27–70.

80. Goetzl EJ, Turck CW, Sreedharan SP. Production and recognition of neuropeptides by cells of the immune system. In: Ader R, Felten DL, Cohen N, ed. Psychoneuroimmunology. San Diego: Academic Press, Inc., 1991: 263–282.

81. Wybran J. Enkephalins and endorphins as modifiers of the immune system: present and future. Federation Proceedings 1985;44:92–94.

82. Goetzl EJ, Sneedham SP. Mediators of communication and adaptation in the neuroendocrine and immune systems. FASEB Journal 1992;6:2646–2652.

83. Goodkin K, Antoni MH, Helder L, Sevin B. Psychoneuroimmunological aspects of disease progression among women with human papillomavirus-associated cervical dysplasia and human immunodeficiency virus type 1 co-infection. International Journal of Psychiatry in Medicine 1993;23:119–148.

84. McGillis JP, Mitsuhashi M, Payan DG. Immunologic properties of Substance P. In: Ader R, Felten DL, Cohen N, ed. Psychoneuroimmunology. San Diego: Academic Press, Inc., 1991: 209–224.

85. Gershon MD, Chalazonitis A, Rothman TP. From neural crest to bowel: development of the enteric nervous system. Journal of Neurobiology 1993;24:199–214.

86. Bockman DE, Kirby ML. The role of the neural crest in the development of the immune system and endocrine organs. In: Freier S, ed. The Neuroendocrine-Immune Network. Boca Raton: CRC Press, Inc., 1990: 1–8.

87. Tse ASD, Barclay N, Watts A, Williams AF. A glycophospholipid tail at the corboxyl terminus of the Thy-1 glycoprotein of neurons and thymocytes. Science 1985;230:1003–1008.

88. Levy JA. Concepts in HIV neuropathogenesis. In: Neu HC, Levy JA, Weiss R, ed. Focus on HIV, 1992. London: Churchill Livingstone, 1993: 51–67.

89. Berczi I, Nagy E. Effects of hypophysectomy on immune function. In: Ader R, Felten DL, Cohen N, ed. Psychoneuroimmunology. San Diego: Academic Press, Inc., 1991: 338–402.

90. Mathews PM, Rooelich CJ, Sibbitt WL, Jr., Bankhurst AD. Enhancement of natural cytotoxicity by beta-endorphin. Journal of Immunology 1983;130:1658.

91. Maestroni GJM, Conti A. The pineal neurohormone melatonin stimulates activated CD4+ Thy-1+ cells to release opioid agonist(s) with immunoenhancing and anti-stress properties. Journal of Neuroimmunology 1990;28:167–176.

92. Krueger JM, Walter J, Dinarello CA, Wolff M, Chedid L. Sleep-promoting effects of endogenous pyrogen (interleukin-1). American Journal of Physiology 1984;246:R994-R999.

93. Darko DF, Miller JC, Gallen C, et al. Sleep electroencephalogram delta-frequency amplitude, night plasma levels of tumor necrosis factor- alpha, and human immunodeficiency virus infection. Proceedings of the National Academy of Sciences (USA) 1995;92:12080–12084.

94. Besedovsky HO, del Rey AE, Sorkin E. Immune-neuroendocrine interactions. Journal of Immunology 1985;135:750s-754s.

95. Koff W, Dunegan MA. Modulation of macrophage-mediated tumoricidal activity by neuropeptides and neurohormones. Journal of Immunology 1985;135:350–354.

96. Blalock JE. The immune system as a sensory organ. Journal of Immunology 1984;132:1067–1070.

97. Blalock JE, Harbour-McMenamin D, Smith EM. Peptide hormones shared by the neuroendocrine and immunologic systems. Journal of Immunology 1985;135:858s–861s.
98. Smith E, Meyer W, Blalock JE. Virus-induced corticosterone in hypophysectomized mice: a possible lymphoid adrenal axis. Science 1982;218:1311.
99. Metal'nikov S, Chorine V. The role of conditioned reflexes in immunity. Annals of the Pasteur Institute 1926;40:893–900.
100. Ader R, Cohen N. Behaviourally conditioned immunosuppression. Psychosomatic Medicine 1975;37:333.
101. Ader R, Cohen N. Behaviourally conditioned immunosuppression and murine systemic lupus erythematosus. Science 1982;214:1534.
102. Bovbjerg D, Ader R, Cohen N. Acquisition and extinction of conditioned suppression of a graft vs. host response in the rat. Journal of Immunology 1984;132:111–113.
103. Ghanta VK, Solvason HB, Hiramoto RN. Augmentation of natural immunity by conditioning and possible mechanisms of enhancement. In: Freier S, ed. The Neuroendocrine-Immune Network. Boca Raton: CRC Press, Inc., 1990: 103–113.
104. Ader R, Cohen N. The influence of conditioning on immune responses. In: Ader R, Felten DL, Cohen N, ed. Psychoneuroimmunology. San Diego: Academic Press, Inc., 1991: 611–646.
105. Olness K, Ader R. Conditioing as an adjunct in the parmacotherapy of lupus erythematosus. Developmental and Behavioral Pediatrics 1992;13:124–125.
106. Cassileth BR, Lusk EJ, Guerry D, et al. Survival and quality of life among patients receiving unproven as compared with conventional cancer therapy. New England Journal of Medicine 1991;324:1180–1185.
107. Weil A. Spontaneous Healing.New York: A. Knopf, 1995

3

THE EVOLUTION OF QUALITY OF LIFE

C. R. B. Joyce

Department of Psychology
Royal College of Surgeons in Ireland
Mercer St
Dublin 2
Ireland

INTRODUCTION

Whole civilisations will have to be ignored in this discussion, for example, classical Chinese, Japanese and Islamic. Each would have provided much relevant material for the three topics of this paper: the definition of Quality of Life; the methodology of its investigation; and changes in Quality of Life itself: past, present and perhaps future.

DEFINITIONS

William James said of consciousness "Its meaning we know so long as no one asks us to define it."[1] This description could equally well apply to Quality of Life, but we need not be so pessimistic as Chardonne: "Rien de précieux n'est transmissible. Une vie heureuse est un secret perdu."[2] More specifically, Quality of Life is (1) what "society" says it is, which is called Health Status, or Health-Related Quality of Life; (2) what the individual says it is; (3) what the individual tells him/herself it is[3] and (4) what his selves argue about. Hundreds of published definitions can be fitted somewhere onto this continuum.

THE PAST

Adam and Eve must have experienced an excellent Quality of Life that has never been as good since they underwent punctate evolution. Recent research strongly suggests that human beings may be descended from a single historical Eve and Adam who lived in Africa between 50 and 400 thousand years [4,5] In a fundamental sense, therefore, all our genes must have some relationship to our Quality of Life, and it is not surprising that many of the elements that enter into its description are common to all of us. Unfortu-

Cancer, AIDS, and Quality of Life, edited by Levy *et al.*
Plenum Press, New York, 1997

nately, this seems to be less true for the more constructive traits than those which seem dominant at present. However, as there is no obvious reason why this should be so, pessimism may be misplaced.

The first published rule for the study of individual Quality of Life was that to be found at the entrance to the Temple of Delphi: "Know thyself !". (Goethe later commented: "If I knew myself, I'd run away !"[6] and Rousseau "I fear the boredom of being alone with myself."[7]) Aristotle defined some components of the Good Life, distinguishing between that of three classes: rulers, warriors and philosophers; but his ideas were generalisations, not personal statements. So were most opinions expressed from classical times until the Renaissance; there were few clear evaluations of factors of personal relevance and none about their relative importance (in modern jargon, their "ratings" and "weights"). The apparent self-revelations of Marcus Aurelius, for example, were really admonitions of others. "A little flesh, a little breath, and a Reason to rule all - that is myself"[8] or "A man should habituate himself to such a way of thinking that if suddenly asked, 'What is in your mind at this minute ?' he could respond frankly and without hesitation..."[8] They have a deceptively modern flavour, but the impersonal tone is clearer when he writes: "Waste no more time arguing what a good man should be. Be one."[8] Other Romans of more epicurean style reveal little more of themselves: "That man is by no means poor, who has the use of everything he wants. If it is well with your belly, your back and your feet, regal wealth can add nothing greater," says Horace;[9] and Martial: "The good man prolongs his life; to be able to enjoy one's past life is to live twice."[10] Marcus Aurelius again: "I often marvel how it is that though each man loves himself beyond all else, he should yet value his own opinion of himself less than that of others."[8] Would he consider this observation valid today ?

Lyric poetry, which originated in Greece in about the seventh century before the Christian era, on the other hand was "short, personal and spoke directly... about individual emotions."[11] But this style was soon buried, and was not disinterred until, much later, the Enlightenment opened the way for the Romantic Movement's convulsive outpourings of personal feelings.

There had probably been little substantive change in Quality of Life itself between Aristotle and Descartes. Technological progress was real, but slow. Its major fruits prepared the way for the later explosion that still continues, but were at first enjoyed only by few. The medical revolution initiated by Pasteur came two hundred years after the Dutch invention of the microscope that made it possible.

Descartes' dictum "Je pense, donc je suis" has long been fair game for philosophical humourists ("Je pense, donc je suis français"), but had he added "I also feel, therefore I am myself twice over", the study of Quality of Life might have started as early as the 17th century. However, Descartes could scarcely have thought such a thought, still less recorded it.

In the eighteenth century sentiments like "Si je ne suis pas meilleur, au moins je suis autre"; or "On dirait que mon coeur et mon esprit n'appartiennent pas au même individu"[12] could at last be uttered again. Self-involvement and the exploration of self began in earnest. The English Critical Ballads, the German Bildungsroman and parallel developments in France and elsewhere described insights into the Quality of Life of their authors. But even such an expanding library of first person accounts could only give a biassed idea of the Quality of Life in general, because the contributors to it were exclusively the literate and articulate -and seldom numerate. Erasmus, rather surprisingly, considered that curiosity "should be restricted to the elite";[7] even so, the systematic study of behaviour did not begin until the middle of the nineteenth century.

Bacon, Hume, Vico, and Lamarck all proposed rules and methods for a science of man according to the ideas about scientific method that prevailed in their own time. The possibility had apparently even been anticipated by Anaximander, Thales and Pythagoras. The earliest English usage of the term "Anthropology" dates from 1593, that of "Evolution" (1830) from nearly 250 years later and of "Sociology" from 1837, following quickly on its coinage by Comte in 1830. The father of each science was ambitious for it to become the science of life, or biology, especially of man.

THE PRESENT

At the midpoint of the nineteenth century, in Susan Sontag's view health began to interest scientists and sickness interested lay people.[13] In the first half of the 20th century, however, sickness began to interest doctors as well, as the physical means of treatment at their disposal evolved. Meanwhile, psychological progress was hindered by its attempts to emulate the methods of the physical sciences. In the mid-1960s medicine began to take a specific interest in physical Quality of Life (the term seems to have been first used by architects some 30 years earlier). In the late 20th century, psychic and physical health have both become of obsessive interest to lay persons. Meanwhile, clinical examination of the outside has yielded to technological examination of the inside of the body, and psychological study of the mind is again giving way to neurological examination of the brain. These developments may be vital to research, and may have improved the health of some who could afford them, but they have distracted attention from the personal significance illness to the affected individual. This bias is fortunately being opposed by the increased interest in individual Quality of Life, especially with the new methods of Gordon Guyatt, Danny Ruta or Ciaran O'Boyle that allow both subject and investigator to look inside the black box.[14]

It is unfortunate that some practitioners in our own culture and, it seems, the majority in other countries, such as Japan or Greece, believe that the Quality of Life of patients with severe or incurable diseases cannot (by which they mean should not) be studied at all. On the contrary, there is evidence that many terminally ill patients welcome such unusual inquiries, as well as the opportunity otherwise denied them to behave altruistically by participating in research. It is as essential to diagnose motivation, which includes the need for information, as it is the disease itself, whatever the culture or the belief system of the family or physician. Indeed, the Quality of Life of many patients may actually be improved by fulfilling their desire to participate in research.[15]

Goethe and Rousseau both alluded to the necessity for honesty, and Goethe, at least, was also aware of the difficulty of achieving it. Lewontin points out that "the pretense is <often> made that problems that cannot be solved are really nothing to worry about... Biologists will apply the most critical and demanding canons of evidence in the design of measuring instruments or in the procedure for taking an unbiased sample," but when the investigators are asked whether the members of that sample are likely to tell the truth about their sexual behaviour, for instance, they "provide a hand-waving intuitive argument filled with unsubstantiated guesses and prejudices."[16]

Questionnaires, the instruments most frequently used for studying so-called Quality of Life, are especially open to this criticism. As Diane Johnson remarks: "We all know that <none of> the choices in the dry language of a questionnaire (Not at all, Very Little, Somewhat, Pretty much, Very much, Don't know)... capture the precise nature of our experience, which is more Sort of, or Pretty much some of the time but sometimes never."[17]

Table 1. Quality of Life scores measured over time

	Scores	GP mean	IND changes	
Pre-Treatment	1 3 4 5 7	4 ± 2.2	—	
Time A	1 3 4 5 7	4 ± 2.2		5 nc
Time B	4 4 4 4 4	4 ± 0.0	2↓2↑	1 nc
Time C	2 0 0 0 0 0	4 ± 8.0	4↓1↑	
Time D	2 4 5 6 3	4 ± 1.6	1↓4↑	

The investigation of Quality of Life has recently begun to escape from such anti-individual tyranny by means of the new methods just mentioned. Nevertheless, epidemiology, sociology and psycho-analysis, all based on the study of groups (unrepresentative though they may sometimes be), still largely dominate the applied behavioural sciences.

The value of the social and individual points of view can be contrasted more sharply. The Table shows hypothetical observations on the Quality of Life of a group of five individuals at baseline and on four successive occasions. The group and individual statistics lead to very different conclusions. The mean score of the group is 4 each time, but is made up in very different ways. Although such group stability may satisfy politicians and hospital directors, it is misleading about individual outcome, and means nothing to the individuals themselves.

IRRELEVANCE OF GROUP STATISTICS TO THE INDIVIDUAL

The distinction is of vital importance because the application of inappropriate social paradigms can compel changes in ways of life that are painful for some people. In 1215, in Britain, the barons extracted from their king the freedom of the Great Charter. In 1996, worldwide, the contemporary barons revolt against their own serfs, extorting economies from the less fortunate; inequality between the top and bottom widens. Typical consequences have been described by Joan Didion as the growth of "... a relatively new kind of monied class... devoid of social responsibility precisely because their ties to any one place had been so attenuated"[18] and "... the creation of an ever-growing pool of unemployable citizens who can neither compete nor consume."[19] A former British Prime Minister seems to have approved of this deplorable situation, for she fashioned from it the political principle that "There is no such thing as society".

Because the pursuit of diametrically opposed and untestable hypotheses about ends and means attracts those who practise the applied social sciences, we may with neither more nor less validity suggest that the comfortable minority could just as well have assumed responsibility for the underprivileged. There has been little evidence of this. In fact, among the side-effects of the evolution of individual Quality of Life is the narcissism that contributes little to society. Judeo-Christian respect for "the irreducible element of divinity in all human beings" - a belief whose value has been heightened "by the terrible human costs of the socialist experiments," according to Genovese, has been gradually perverted, and has become "an ignoble dream of personal liberation;" whether "in its radical-democratic, communist or free-market form, <it has> proven the most dangerous illusion of our time."[20]

THE FUTURE

It may be difficult to analyse the past and impossible to describe the present, but it is certainly foolhardy to predict the future, as the promises of politicians and the recipes of economists show. However, two forecasts seem safe, although not entirely uncontested: population in non-western countries will continue to increase, as will the economic gap between rich and poor, for individuals as well as countries.

Less certainly, the control of Quality of Life will become more systematic, not only by genetic manipulation, but also by Orwellian vocabulary control (such as "welfare reform" instead of "welfare destruction" and "downsizing" instead of "massive firings"). On the positive side, programmes for monitoring personal Quality of Life will serve increased opportunities for leisure, helping to plan the individual's life and monitoring progress towards the attainment of personal objectives. These factors, with the broader social relationships made possible by modern technology, such as the increasing application of Virtual Reality, could reduce pressure on personal space, and so cut down displays of aggression.

Among the many that weave their way through human behaviour, however, the cyclical pattern of compassion to heartlessness is now sweeping decisively towards the callous. A recent survey found that Australians experience anger five times more often than sympathy. But the form of the question may affect answers: probing about "self-sacrifice" instead of asking about "giving of oneself" reduced the number of American altruists by over 60%.[7]

Prolonging life will still be thought worthwhile, despite falling birth rates in some countries and high child mortality in others, and aging populations will demand funds for research upon aging. (The belief that aging is a disease seems to imply that life itself is inherently unhealthy.) A better strategy would enable the young to earn higher wages sooner. The contemporary enactment of this strategy is not only more apparent than real: it is partial and irrelevant, applying primarily to mainly non-productive professions such as stockbroking, public relations and the manufacture of armaments. Enterprising insurance agents will explicitly encourage the wealthy to insure themselves against deterioration in their Quality of Life; it is unlikely in the present climate that social security programmes will be able to insure the majority. The ease with which much of the diminishing amount of work still to be performed by human beings can be carried out at home, by men as well as women, already affects the Quality of Life of whole families. Men, too, are becoming accessible to the demands of all members of the family.

Now to pure speculation: the acquisition of religious experiences without recourse to organised religion or hallucinogenic drugs will become easier; the monitoring of dream content will make possible the control of dreaming by others as well as ourselves, and dream libraries will be developed that allow us to rerun our own dreams, and to borrow those of others. It is a moot point whether all these developments will lead to increased individual creativity, but it will become possible to estimate Quality of Life continuously. Catheters or electrodes might be routinely inserted at birth into the frontal lobes or third ventricle.

If ethical behaviour is subject to evolutionary development and there is still time for moral behaviour to be reselected the human race may yet survive.

THE THIRD WORLD

The homogeneity implied in the concept is of course absurd. But it has been estimated that 90% of the between four and six thousand living world languages will probably disappear within the next hundred years, as part of the "general loss being suffered by the world, the loss of diversity in all things."

The serious study of Quality of Life is likely to remain as much a Northern-, First-World luxury as at present. (A recent document from a well-known international organisation equated the quality of one western life with that of fifteen Third World lives, confusing quality with their value, and being wrong about both.) It is often implied that the Third World does not suffer from chronic diseases (presumably because its inhabitants do not live long enough to get them), but it is true that chronic misery is even more widespread than chronic disease.

Many investigators living in the so-called First World believe that the components of Quality of Life of different cultures are surprisingly similar. Such complacency has at least three origins. Mention has already been made of the first two of these: failure to distinguish between group and individual; the deficiencies of questionnaire-based investigations. The third is the confusion between the dimensions of Quality of Life and the factors that contribute to them. These enter into the generally accepted dimensions: Cognitive, Affective, Social, Physical and Ecological. A philosophical, spiritual or Religious dimension is more and more found to be necessary (CASPER). It is these dimensions that are common to cultures and individuals. The conceptual factors that enter into them differ.

However, there is little more than anecdotal evidence from which to conclude that the Quality of Life of a single Haitian, Cambodian, Rwandan or inhabitant of the country that was once called both Falastina and Eretz Israel is either satisfactory or unsatisfactory as intuition often suggests. Two hundred years ago, Captain Cook was an early optimist about the Hawaiians: "They may appear to some to be the most wretched people upon the earth; but in reality they are far happier than we Europeans."[21] A modern insider witness, the South African musician Hugh Masekela, agrees that "Despite all the oppression, <we> are the happiest people I've ever known... the European mind-set has always been rather annoyed about how <the enslaved> people still have a better time than they do... the oppressor says 'How come they're laughing and I'm so miserable ?'"[22] Third World appearances and structures are not only to be found in the so-called "Third World" itself, but also in sub-cultures of rich and evolved societies. The American poetess Nikki Giovanni hopes "no white person has cause to write about me because... they'll probably talk about my very hard childhood and never understand that all the while I was quite happy."[23] Paul Feyerabend thinks that the !Kung "survive happily... in surroundings where any Western person would come in and die after a few days. But the question is, What is the quality of life ? And that has not been decided."[24]

CONCLUSION

Health Status and Quality of Life are not opposed but complementary. However, whereas the methodologies for their study are steadily improving, the actual Quality of Life of many, perhaps the majority of individuals and peoples has worsened. The decision to smoke, use drugs or exercise a sexual preference is finally an individual matter, but genetic, social and environmental factors enter into each. The early anecdotal information came from qualitative individual accounts by literate individuals. That we can now study the Health Status of large numbers quantitatively should not cause us to lose sight of the enduring importance of the Quality of individual lives, literate and less literate, rich and poor, and healthy as well as sick.

Three hundred years later Pablo Neruda, too, updated Descartes: "Pronuncio y soy."[25] A single word cannot retranslate the Spanish into either Latin or French. "Pronuncio" encompasses not only speaking, oration, declamation, but even judgment - and also action.

ACKNOWLEDGMENTS

Professors H-U Fisch and Anna Wirz-Justice, and Drs B Hiltbrunner, I Kostaki and N Palmer very helpfully criticised an earlier and fuller draft.

REFERENCES

1. James W. The Principles of Psychology, Vol 1.New York:Dover,1950.
2. Chardonne J. Claire. Paris:Grasset, 1931.
3. Joyce CRB. How can we measure individual quality of life ? Schweizerische Medizinische Wochenschrift 1995;124:1921–1926.
4. Hammer MF. A recent common ancestry for human Y chromosomes. Nature 1995;378:376–378.
5. Whitfield IS, Sulston JE and Goodfellow PN. Sequence variation of the human Y chromosome. Nature 1995;378:379–380.
6. Goethe JW von. In: Auden WH and Kronenberger L, eds. The Viking Book of Aphorisms. A Personal Selection. New York:Viking,1962.
7. Zeldin T. An Intimate History of Humanity. London:Minerva,1995.
8. Marcus Aurelius. Meditations. London:Penguin 1995.
9. Horace. Epistle XII: To Iccius.
10. Martial. Epigrams Book X 23.
11 Balmer J. Sappho: Poems and Fragments. Newcastle-upon-Tyne: Bloodaxe Books, 1992.
12. Rousseau J-J. Oeuvres Complètes. Vol 1. Paris: Bibliothèque de la Pleiade, 1959.
13. Sontag S. Illness as Metaphor. London:Allan Lane, 1979.
14. O'Boyle C, McGee H and Joyce CRB, eds. Chur: Harcourt. In preparation.
15. Feenberg A. On being a human subject: interest and obligation in the experimental treatment of human disease. Philosophical Forum 1992;23:213–230.
16. Lewontin RC. Sex, Lies and Social Science (Review of *The Social Organization of Sexuality: Sexual practices in the United States*. Laumann EO, Gagnon JH, Michael RT and Michaels S. Chicago: UCP, 1995). New York Review, 1995 April 20:24–29.
17. Johnson D. New York Review 1989, Oct 12:25–27.
18. Didion J. Sentimental Journeys. London:Harper Collins, 1993.
19. Davis DB. Southern Comfort. Review of three books by Eugene D Genovese. New York Review. 1995, Oct 5:43–46.
20. Quoted by Davis DB, *op cit.*
21. Cook J. In: Clark M. A Short History of Australia. Ringwood, Victoria:Penguin,1986.
22. Masekela H interviewed by Mike Zwerin, International Herald Tribune 1992,July 23.
23. Giovanni N. Nikki Rosa. In: Toni Cade, ed. The Black Woman. New York: New American Library, 1970.
24. Feyerabend P interviewed by John Horgan: Scientific American, May 1993.
25. Neruda P. La Palabra (from Plenos Poderes, 1962). In: Tarn N, ed. Pablo Neruda. Selected Poems. London: Penguin, 1975.

4

QUALITY OF CARE FOR CANCER AND AIDS

Robert J. D. George

Palliative Care Center
Department of Psychiatry and Behavioural Science
UCL Medical School and
Camden and Islington Community Health Services NHS Trust
Palliative Care Team
London, United Kingdom

INTRODUCTION

This paper addresses the Quality of Care that we provide for patients, and see how it relates to Quality of Life (QoL). Clearly any health care that is provided for the individual must have as its basic motivation the restoration of that person as near to full health as possible. In the case of my own specialty, the care of the dying, this is of course not possible, and endeavours in that direction are fruitless. *Our* measurement of Care Outcome, therefore, can not have a defined clinical endpoint such as cure, but must rather turn to facets of the individual that have been favourably influenced by our interventions. This will of course include clinical factors such as symptom control. Unless we are able to demonstrate improvement in our patients, and for the benefit of our funders provide some kind of measurement, we are not in a position to defend what we do, or to claim that work is of value. With respect to all patients, but the dying in particular, QoL is of the essence, and should be the predominent motivation that our management has in driving it.

In order to explore the relationships between QoL, Quality of Care and our Care Outcomes, it is necessary to simplify the "construct" of QoL quite substantially. Their complexity is, in many ways, the dominating component of this Conference. However, the formulations that we explore should establish, in principle at least, how we should configure our care packages, the services that we provide and the benchmarks that define Standards of Care. I will explore these concepts using a graphical representation of the factors, and offer some quasi formulae.[1] We will begin by providing some basic breakdown of QoL in the dying, and how this should inform our Philosophy of Care. We will then move on to consider Care Outcome and how that may be formulated, look at a possible methodology for measuring these, and finally explore how changes in these factors are likely to influence the service we provide.

Cancer, AIDS, and Quality of Life, edited by Levy *et al.*
Plenum Press, New York, 1997

QUALITY OF LIFE

One may reasonably suggest that each of us has aspirations that define what we consider to be a perfect life. These are often nebulous things, but within Palliative Care and Care of the Dying, they fall into three broad categories:

- those relating to the *physical*, such as goals within our profession or physical activities - an example would be to reach as high a standard as possible in a chosen task, be that within leisure and employment;
- matters relating to our *emotions* and psyche such as the nature and quality of our relationships with family, partner and friends,
- some expression of our perception of the world and how we fit into it with respect to purpose - the so called *existential or spiritual* domain.

These interact together to provide us with meaning and a sense of self. For the dying, this global perception is of the essence and each domain may affect significantly QoL and a peaceful death. The social domain is addressed briefly below.

Figure 1 illustrates their relationship very simply. Think of three concentric spheres lying within each other, much as an egg or a Russian doll:

The central one represents the existential or spiritual - ones being. The shell lying outside that represents the emotional and psychological - feeling, and the outermost shell, the physical or doing. Optimum balances between these three broad areas might add together to provide what we could call aspiration, or our contemporary sense of perfection. Not surprisingly the individual components of this will vary with time in their significance: for example a newborn child is interested in little other than eating, sleeping and excreting, whereas the young man is pre-occupied with the physical and periodically the emotional, and the older person is more "philosophical": considering matters of meaning, integration of the past and the more transcendent view to be more appropriate thoughts.

One's achievements are, of course, the degrees to which one fulfils these aspirations, and are, therefore, a function of spiritual/existential and emotional health, and physical capability.

Each of these components of achievement over time is added, and the closeness with which they reach our aspirations may reasonably be said to represent how close we are to perfection, and therefore to reflect our QoL. More precisely, that quality is to be reflected in the degree to which our achievements fall short of aspiration, in other words, it is a function of the *aspiration–achievement gap*. The smaller that this is, the closer and better is our QoL to perfection. This concept can be expressed mathematically as a reciprocal relationship.

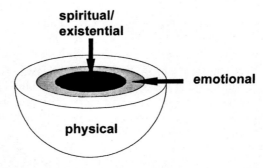

Figure 1. The Egg. A symbolic model of the three personal elements that are relevant in the care of the dying.

$$QoL \; \alpha \; \frac{1}{[ASPIRATION] - [ACHIEVEMENT]} \tag{1}$$

where:

ASPIRATION = *f [goals, relationships, world view, meaning, sense of self]*

ACHIEVEMENT = *f [spiritual/existential and emotional health, physical* capability*]*

This idea is expressed graphically in Figure 2. The Time line runs from adolescence through illness to death. On this graph, with the passage of time, the dominance of the physical part of life in youth inevitably changes because of one's declining strength, and is replaced and compensated for by greater emphasis on the emotional and ultimately the existential as death approaches. Note also on this figure that the interrupted line represents the limit of acceptable QoL. Should our overall QoL fall below this, then we will register it eg "life is aweful", "I can't go on like this" etc. The central dip represents life-threatening illness, following which physical capabilities decline, and ultimately one dies.

Figure 3, presents the three components of QoL separated out on a background of the total measurement of achievement. It shows more clearly how each domain may change both with time and in response to circumstances. The time from the onset of fatal disease is shown in Figure 4. However, in this figure, the three domains are separated out, and expressed as positive or negative changes from the time of the onset of fatal disease: thus each starts at zero. The point of particular relevance is that the line representing the physical gradually decreases and might be seen in isolation as less and less acceptable (namely a negative figure), yet the lines representing the psychological and the spiritual/existential are increasing substantially, both in absolute terms and in percentage.

In summary, then, the true measurement of QoL may be said to be the gap between aspiration and achievement, which in themselves are quite difficult things to measure. QoL is normally expressed indirectly by measuring components of achievement, namely by physical capability, emotional and existential health. They are, however, seldom equated with aspiration, and to my knowledge never expressed exlicitly as a relationship. This is important, since with the passage of time, changes in a person's situation, such as the threat of death, intuitively mean a fall in QoL. Yet this can be restored into the acceptable range by focussing on the non-physical dimensions of care. The loss from declining physical capabilities may be substituted very effectively with improved psychological health and well being by attending to questions of meaning, existence and the spiritual.

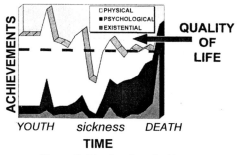

Figure 2. The domains of achievement.

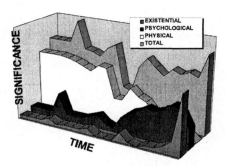

Figure 3. The domain plots of Quality of Life.

These last two areas may increase very substantially compared with their baseline importance or relevance at the time the patient first presented with illness and they can lead to vistors and depths of experience opening for the first time in a person's life.

It is worth making two additional points. Firstly, I have left the social dimensions of quality out for reasons of simplicity. They are naturally very important and in many respects form part of the physical adjustments that will minimise the difficulties of incapacity. I refer here to things such as accomodation, practical aids, financial support and practical assistance from informal or paid carers. Secondly, I have made the assumption that Aspiration is a fixed thing. Clearly it is not. For example, the expectations from life of a hopeful, ambitious youngster compared with their perceptions of what makes a life worth living decades later are radically different. To be pedantic, therefore, the line of Aspiration will fluctuate with time as does Achievement. However, I have taken that to be self evident and for simplicity represented aspiration as a constant ceiling in these discussions.

QUALITY OF LIFE AND ITS INFLUENCE ON PHILOSOPHY OF CARE AND CARE PROVISION

It now seems logical that in configuring the care we offer, the nature and character of an individual's QoL and the ways in which we can improve it productively should be central in informing us of how to go about things. This formulation is classically ex-

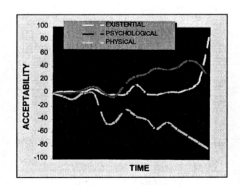

Figure 4. Quality of Life: Changing priorities over time.

pressed in the Philosophy of Care that a service expresses and holds to. For example, in the service we provide in the UK, our motives are to minimise the physical discomfort and problems around the dying process, focus clinical care on fulfulling realistic practical tasks, and as it were reduce the negative aspects of physical deterioration to a minimum; psychologically to work very positively with the patient and family to optimise relationship, and give the individual an opportunity to explore questions related to the meaning of their life, and what may lie beyond death. This is expressed as follows:

"Palliative Care should incorporate and integrate the best in physical, social, psychological and spiritual care. We aim to give optimum pain and symptom control at all stages of illness. We aim also to allow patients and caregivers to prepare for death within a framework and worldview of their choice. The overall objective is to provide a safe and suitable environment for the individual to complete tasks and examine areas in which there may be conflict or concern. This must:

- *be clinically, psychologically, culturally and spiritually appropriate*
- *respect the autonomy of patients in determining the nature and course of their care*
- *be able to accommodate change*
- *be neutral - having the capacity to inform and assist patients in decision making, without bias*

Success depends on effective multi-disciplinary practice. In the interests of patients and professionals, there must be mechanisms for clear, confidential communication amongst practitioners and with their clients. Mutual respect, understanding and support where problems arise in dealing with difficult or complex situations are essential."

Following from this we configure care individually such that its quality seeks to optimise and reach the philosophy.

In a broad sense, our *Philosophy of Care is our Aspiration*, and the *Quality of Care we provide is our Achievement*, paralleling the formulation of QoL.

Whilst we would define minimum standards of care below which our Service is unacceptable, and above which we are achieving our goals, this Quality of Care will, of course, be influenced not only by Philosophy of Practice and the configuration of Service that we deliver, but also by Local and National Policy, the availability of resources, the involvement of allied professionals and colleagues, and the partnership with the patient (ie their autonomy). This is a simple function:

Quality of Care = f[Philosophy of Care, Service, Health Priority, Patient Autonomy] (2)

FORMULATING THE CARE OUTCOME

We now have some idea of how to come up with some measurement of QoL - albeit expressed indirectly through Achievements, though ideally referenced internally to the patient and their Aspirations.

We are referred a patient at a given point, when QoL may be at a nadir. It is then our task to provide a service that optimises this QoL over time, and ideally ends with a patient dying with as much sense of health and personal well-being as they had prior to diagnosis, if not better. Implicitly this involves the collaboration and choice of the patient insofar as we can merely offer services, we cannot force them upon individuals.

This concept is expressed in Figure 5. The curve of the change in QoL following referral demonstrates an improvement and a passing of the threshhold of acceptability over time. This is, of course, a function both of QoL and the patient's choice in allowing service. Our point of referral could be called *Quality of Care₀ (QC₀)* where no Quality of Care has been provided by the service prior to referral and *Quality of Care*$_{MAX}$ *(QC* $_{MAX}$*)* is the best service that we are able to provide:

$$Quality\ of\ care = \int_{QC_0}^{QC_{MAX}} \left[(QoL)(patient\ choice) \right] - (QoL)$$

$$(3)$$

We are now in a position, having constructed a relationship between QoL, and Quality of Care to give us a Care Outcome. These relationships are expressed in Figure 6 and show a familiar cycle of interconnections between Philosophy of Care, service and standards and care outcome. This interrelationship is known otherwise as the *Audit Loop*. We aspire to a task, we provide a service and define the minimum standards for that. This should then be monitored and audited by measuring our care outcomes. For example, if the care outcome falls short of the defined minimum standard, then we are required to optimise the service to reach that, or else address the more fundamental question of whether our Philosophy of Care is actually correct.

$$[Care\ Outcome] = \int_{QC_0}^{QC_{MAX}} \left[(QoL)(patient\ choice) \right] - [QoL]$$

$$(4)$$

where:

QC_0 precedes care and QC_{MAX} is your best service. Hence:

Care outcome > 0 = GOOD
Care outcome < 0 = BAD.

If our care outcome demonstrates improvement, then this should be related not only to Philosophy of Care but also to our construction of the individual, and should be directed at maximising those needs as defined broadly in clinical practice, our construction of the physical, emotional and spiritual elements that are presented to us.

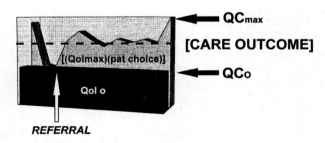

Figure 5. Formulating the care outcome.

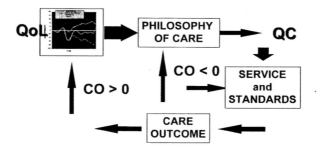

Figure 6. Quality of Care and Audit.

THE COMPONENTS OF CARE OUTCOME

Having established the nature of the work required to achieve our Care Outcome's, we can now break these down into their component tasks. Figure 7 shows two key areas: practical and clinical work, and the psychospiritual work. This requires a spectrum of discipline - such as medicine, nursing, psychological care, dietetics, occupational therapy and trained home carers for those who need 24 hour supervision or basic nursing care at home.

Most of the practical and clinical work is done at the onset of care when symptomatology comes under control, and the environment is optimized. The amount of this input may then decline, and then subsequently rise again towards a time of death when an additional amount of practical help may be required. Psychosocial and spiritual work conversely develops with time following the development of relationship and trust, and this becomes increasingly prominent as death approaches.

MEASUREMENTS OF CARE OUTCOME

Can we measure these theoretical considerations? In short we can, although our current tools are relatively indirect though developing. In our Service, we use a multi-faceted real-time scoring system known as the Support Team Assessment Schedule, which incorporates within it both measurements of Quality of Care and Quality of Life (Fig 8). A detailed analysis of the tool used can be found elsewhere.[2] Using this technique we are able to produce curves of patient care with the passage of time, which appear very similar to the figures given in this paper, and provide some validity to the analysis.

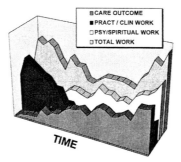

Figure 7. Components of care outcome.

■ **"QUALITY OF CARE"**   ■ **"QUALITY OF LIFE"**
  measure what we claim   *partial measures*

- practical needs   – pain
- finance   – symptoms
- wasted time   – anxiety
- communication   – insight
- advice   – relationships
- location   – spiritual

Figure 8. The components of STAS.

We are currently developing a more sophisticated software tool utilising STAS and detailed measurements of clinical activity, which will allow us to give a complex analysis of the relationship between the QoL, complexity of a case and the nature and type of care that is required.

CONCLUSION

Factors Influencing Care Provision

Having given a broad analysis applying the role of QoL in care provision of the dying, one area remains: the influence that patients, colleagues and resources have on the Quality of Care that we provide.

In Figure 9, the first column on the left shows a minimum of standard of care which should be dependent exclusively upon the resources within the Service, and the contribution of colleagues to that care provision. For example, with respect to cancer, the work of oncologists or radiotherapists. You will see that between the minimum standard and optimum level of care is the component provided by the patient. This acknowledges the individual's autonomy in limiting or having some control over the care provision that he or she receives. The other two columns express the consequences of reduced resources.

- The influence of reduced resources on the core service provision with much of the slack taken up by additional work by colleagues. In this situation, which of course

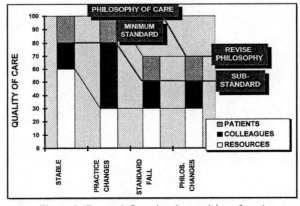

Figure 9. Factors influencing the provision of service.

is implicitly dependent upon good will and commitment of other clinicians to the philosophy of care, the minimum standard is maintained despite a cut in resources.

- Two scenarios where our colleagues are unable to increase their contribution to care. For example, as a result of their own financial constraints in the first maintaining the previous quality of the Philosophy of Care. the only consequence can be the reduction of the minimum standards of care to sub-standard levels.

One is left with simple alternatives. Either a service where the minimum standard is not reached, staff morale is poor and patients expectations are unmet, or an adjustment with a revision of philosophy. This fiscal pressure is for many a reality, despite its unacceptibility. Thus two points can be emphasised:

1. Without an adequate justification of one's Philosophy of Care, it would be difficult to justify any level of resource. The point of this paper.
2. Despite adequate justification, in the face of shrinking budgets a Philosophy of Care may be maintained by extending roles to professionals outside a single service, or alternatively facing the fact that standards will be lower than those which one wishes, or a Philosophy of Care that is suboptimal.

However, should the last event prevail, at least one can be clear that any reduction in budget will be made in the knowledge that the service to patients may suffer.

REFERENCES

1. Calman KC. Quality of Life in Cancer patients - an hypothesis. J Med Ethics 1984 (10) 124 - 127.
2. Higginson I (Ed). Clinical Audit in Palliative Care. Pub Radcliffe Medical Press, Oxford 1993.

5

CHANGING OUR METAPHORS TO PUT QUALITY OF LIFE AT THE CENTER OF HEALTH CARE

George J. Annas

Health Law Department
Boston University Schools of Medicine
  and Public Health
80 E. Concord St.
Boston, Massachusetts 02118

Metaphors matter, as America's defunct health insurance financing debate so well demonstrated. In that debate the traditional metaphor of American medicine, the military metaphor, was displaced in public discourse by the market metaphor. Metaphors, which entice us to understand and experience "one kind of thing in terms of another . . . play a central role in the construction of social and political reality."[1] The market metaphor proved virtually irresistible in the public arena, and led Congress to defer to market forces to "reform" health insurance financing in America.

The United States is a country founded on the proposition that we are all endowed by our creator with certain inalienable rights, especially the rights to life, liberty and the pursuit of happiness. Any government-sponsored health care plan must account for the reality that Americans assume these rights support entitlement. Perhaps as importantly, we live in a wasteful, technologically-driven, individualistic, and death-denying culture. Every health plan, government-sponsored or not, must also take these postmodern American characteristics into account. How is it even possible to think seriously about reforming a health care system that reflects these primal and pervasive American values and characteristics? How is it possible for Americans to begin to take seriously an intuitively shared belief that quality of life is more important than quantity of life? I believe the first necessary step, which will require us to look deeper than money and means, to goals and ends, is to engage a new metaphor to frame our public policy discussion by helping us develop a new conception of health care. We have tried the military metaphor and the market metaphor; both narrow our field of vision and neither can take us where we need to go.

Cancer, AIDS, and Quality of Life, edited by Levy *et al.*
Plenum Press, New York, 1997

THE MILITARY METAPHOR

The military metaphor has had the most pervasive influence over both the practice and financing of medicine in the US, especially in the areas of cancer and AIDS. [23] Nor is the pervasiveness of this metaphor limited to the US. Examples are legion. Medicine is a battle against death. Diseases attack the body, physicians intervene. We are almost constantly engaged in wars on various of these diseases, most notably cancer. Physicians, who are mostly specialists backed by allied health professionals, and trained to be aggressive, fight these invading diseases with various weapons, designed to knock them out. Physicians give orders in the trenches and on the front lines, use their armamentaria in search of breakthroughs. Treatments are conventional or heroic, and the brave patients soldier it out. We engage in triage in the emergency department, invasive procedures in the operating theatre, and even in defensive medicine when a legal enemy is suspected.

The military metaphor leads us to overmobilize and to think of medicine in terms that have become dysfunctional. For example, it encourages us to ignore costs, and leads hospitals and physicians to engage in medical arms races. It tempts us to believe that all problems can be solved with more sophisticated technology. It leads us to accept as inevitable organizations that are hierarchical and male-dominated. It suggests that seeing the patient's body as a battlefield is appropriate, as are short-term, single-minded tactical goals. Military thinking concentrates on the physical, sees control as central, and willingly expends massive resources to achieve dominance.

As pervasive as the military metaphor is in medicine, the metaphor itself has been so sanitized that it is virtually unrelated to the reality of war itself . We have not, for example, used it to assert that medicine, like war, should only be financed and controlled by the government. Nor have we taken the Nuremberg Code seriously enough to insist on strict rules of human experimentation and penalties for those who violate the human rights of their subjects. And the metaphor itself has become mythic.[4] As historian of war, John Keegan, correctly argues, modern warfare has become so horrible that "it is scarcely possible anywhere in the world today to raise a body of reasoned support for the opinion that war is a justifiable activity."[5]

THE MARKET METAPHOR

The market metaphor has already transformed the way we in the US describe and think about fundamental relationships in medical care, but is just as dysfunctional as the military metaphor. In the language of the market, for example, health plans and hospitals market products to consumers who purchase them based on price. Medical care is a business that necessarily involves marketing through advertising and competition among suppliers who see profit making as their primary motivation. Health care becomes managed care. Mergers and acquisitions become core activities. Chains are developed, vertical integration pursued, and antitrust concerns proliferate. Consumer choice becomes the central mantra of the market metaphor.[6] In the language of insurance, consumers become "covered lives" (or even "money-generating biological structures"[7]). economists become health financing gurus. The role of physicians is radically altered as they are instructed by managers that they can no longer be patient advocates (but rather must advocate for the entire group of covered lives in the health plan). In the language of the insurance industry, the provision of medical care becomes a "loss," and is thus to be minimized or avoided altogether if possible. The goal of medicine becomes a healthy bottom line instead of a healthy population.

The market metaphor leads us to think about medicine in already familiar ways: emphasis is placed on efficiency, profit maximization, customer satisfaction, ability to pay, planning, entreprenurship and competitive models. The ideology of medicine is displaced by the ideology of the marketplace.[89] Trust is replaced by *caveat emptor*. There is no place for the poor and uninsured in the market model. Business ethics supplants medical ethics as the practice of medicine becomes corporatized. Nonprofit medical organizations tend to be corrupted by adopting the values of their for profit competitors. A management degree becomes as important, if not more important, than a medical degree. Public institutions, by definition, cannot compete in the for-profit arena, and risk demise, second-class status, or are simply privatized.

Like the mythologized military metaphor, the market metaphor is also a myth. Consumer-patients are to make decisions, but these are now relegated to corporate entities. The market metaphor conceals inherent market imperfections, the medical commons, and the inability of the market to distribute goods and services whose supply and demand is unrelated to price. It pretends that there is such a thing as a free market in health insurance plans, and that purchasers can and should be content with their choices when an unexpected injury or illness strikes them or a family member. The reality is that American markets are highly regulated, major industries enjoy large public subsidies, industrial organizations tend to oligopoly, and strong consumer protection laws and consumer access to the courts to pursue product liability suits are essential to prevent profits from being too ruthlessly pursued.

THE CLINTONS' MIXED METAPHORS

This summary of American medicine's two dominant metaphors helps explain why the Clintons were never able to articulate a coherent view of their goals for a reformed health care financing system. The Clinton plan was said by the President and First Lady to rest on six pillars (or to be guided by six "shining stars"): security, savings, choice, simplicity, responsibility, and quality. These six characteristics mix the military and market metaphors in impossible and inconsistent ways, and add new, unrelated concepts to them as well. The predominant metaphor of the Clintons seems to have been the military one: security was goal number one. But in a post-cold war era, security ("Health care that will always be there") as a reason to make major change is a tough sell. Even harder was selling the health care alliances that were the centerpiece of the new security arrangement. The military metaphor (undercut by words like savings and choice), simply could not provide a coherent vision of the Clinton plan.

Nor could the market metaphor. The key concept to the market is, of course, consumer choice, and this was promised. However, the Clinton plan was founded on choice of health care plan, not choice of physician or treatment, and when the latter choices were seen as central (by Harry and Louise, for example, who said of government health care, "They chose, we lose") the plan itself collapsed, and the alliances with it. Choice, quality, and even savings can be generated by a market plan; but such an approach has little room for either responsibility or simplicity - ecology-related goals that have generated little enthusiasm among contemporary Americans. In retrospect, the Clinton vision seems to have been doomed from the day its six inconsistent foundational principles, goals, or guides were articulated.

The Clintons also failed to engage the four deep-seated negative characteristics of American culture that dominate medical care. Of special note is our denial of death. In perhaps the best response to the successful Harry and Louise campaign against their proposal, the Clintons taped a parody for the annual Gridiron Dinner. The centerpiece was the following dialog between them:

HILLARY . . . On page 12, 743...no, I got that wrong. Its Page 27, 655; it says that eventually we are all going to die.

BILL: Under the Clinton Health Plan? (*Hillary nods gravely*) You mean that after Bill and Hillary put all those new bureaucrats and taxes on us, we're still going to die?

HILLARY: Even Leon Panetta.

BILL: Wow, that *is* scary! I've never been so frightened in all my life!

HILLARY: Me neither, Harry. (*They face the camera*)

BILL & HILLARY: There's *got* to be a better way.[10]

Some commentators, like ABC's Sam Donaldson reacted by stating that you can't discuss death in political discourse and have it help your cause. The Clintons apparently agreed, and the White House decided to refuse to release copies of the videotape of the spoof even for educational use (and even though it had been played on national TV), adopting another leaf from military metaphor by treating it as a top secret document.

It seems reasonable to conclude that if Congress is ever to make meaningful progress on reforming our fast-changing medical care finance and delivery system, a new way must be found to think about health itself. This will require at least a new metaphorical framework that permits us to re-envision and thus to reconstruct America's medical care system; and place much more emphasis on quality of life and prevention, rather than quantity of life and high-tech rescue medicine. I suggest that the leading candidate for this metaphorical replacement is the ecology metaphor.

THE ECOLOGY METAPHOR

Ecologists use words like integrity, balance, natural, limited (resources) , quality (of life), diversity, renewable, sustainable, responsibility (for future generations), community, and conservation.[11] The concepts embedded in these words and others common to the ecology movement, could, if applied to medicine, have a profound impact on the way the debate about it is conducted and on plans for change that are seen as reasonable.

The ecology metaphor could, for example, help us confront and accept limits (both on the expected length of our lives, and the amount of resources we think reasonable to spend to increase longevity), to value nature, and to emphasize quality of life. It could lead us to worry about our grandchildren and thus to plan long term, to favor sustainable technologies over ones that we cannot afford to provide to all who could benefit from them, to emphasize prevention and public health measures, to debate the merits of rationing, and to accept the function of responsible gatekeepers to the medical commons.

Using the ecological (sometimes referred to as the environmental metaphor) is not unprecedented in medicine. Two physician writers, for example, used it extensively. Lewis Thomas often invoked it in his essays in the *New England Journal of Medicine*, and his idea that the earth itself could best be thought of as a "single cell" became the title for his first collection of these essays, *The Lives of a Cell*.[12] Using this metaphor helped him, I think, to develop many of his important insights related to modern medicine, including the concept of a "halfway technology, his arguments that death should not be seen as the enemy, and that in viewing humans as part of the environment we could see ourselves in a new perspective, as highly specialized handymen (sic) for the earth: "Who knows, we might even acknowledge the fragility and vulnerability that always accompany high specialization in biology, and movements might start up for the protection of ourselves as a valuable, endangered species. We couldn't lose."[12]

The other leading physician spokesperson for an ecological view of medicine is Van Renselaer Potter, who in coining the term "bioethics" in 1971 meant it to apply not just to medical ethics (its contemporary meaning) but to a blend of biological knowledge and human values that took special account of environmental values.[13] In his words, "Today we need biologists who respect the fragile web of life and who can broaden their knowledge to include the nature of man and his (sic) relation to the biological and physical worlds."[13]

Drawing on the attempts of the "deep ecologists" to ask more fundamental questions than their "shallow" environmental counterparts (who concentrate on pollution abatement),[14] psychiatrist Willard Gaylin fruitfully suggested that the Clinton approach to health care reform was itself shallow.[15] He correctly, I think, suggested that what was needed was a "wide-open far-ranging public debate about the deeper issues of health care - our attitudes toward life and death, the goals of medicine, the meaning of health, suffering versus survival, who shall live and who shall die (and who shall decide)..."[15] Without addressing these deeper questions Gaylin rightly argues, we can never solve our health care crisis.

An ecological metaphor also naturally leads to considerations of population health rather than concentration solely on the health of individuals. In this sense, medicine becomes a subset of public health, rather than the other way around. It leads away from concentration on individual risk factors, for example, "toward the social structures and processes within which ill-health originates, and which will often be more amenable to modification."[16] Using an ecological metaphor, it leads us to look "upstream" (reference to another metaphor about villagers who devised even more complex technologies to save people from drowning, rather than looking upstream to see who was pushing them in.) to see what is causing the downstream illnesses and injuries.[17] It leads us to put much more emphasis on prevention and public health interventions, and less on wasteful end-of-life interventions.[18] In short, quality of life becomes much more important than quantity of life.

Although the market has already proven destructive in the US, perhaps it is not to unrealistic to see the current surge of market medicine as a forest fire: we used to believe fire only destroyed nature, but now we know that its role is much more subtle, including burning off of "dead wood" and the release of seeds and changing habitat for new species to flourish. Perhaps the fire of market medicine presages a similar change for the better in the American health care system.

CONTROL AND CONFORMITY

The dominance in our thinking about medicine by the military and market metaphors has reinforced two quests that seem to define both modern medicine and postmodern politics: quests for control and conformity. Control of nature, of course, remains contemporary medicine's primary goal, and its accomplishments have been astonishing at both borders of life. Medical technology has, for example, eliminated the necessity to engage in sexual intercourse to procreate, and in the process radically altered the meaning of parenthood in ways we have yet to confront socially. At life's other border, we continue our quest to banish death - and if that cannot be done, control is asserted in the name of freedom to end life itself. The quest for conformity may seem an anomaly in a society of individualists, but physicians know better. Cosmetic surgery designed to sculpt bodies to conform to a socially-constructed ideal of healthy has become a major industry. Mind-altering drugs promise mental conformity, and new drugs, such as human growth hormone, promise at least a degree of physical conformity. The human genome project promises even more: that we will understand and be able to manipulate our genes in a way that makes our current surgical and chemical manipulations of human characteristics seem primitive.

By valuing diversity and rejecting complete control of nature as a reasonable goal, the ecological metaphor may help us reexamine our commitments to control and conformity in medicine. Unlike the military and market metaphors as well, which only reinforce our counterproductive American characteristics of wastefulness, technology obsession, fear of death, and individualism, the ecological metaphor could help us to confront them. The ecological metaphor in medicine can encourage an alternative vision of resource conservation, sustainable technologies, acceptance of death as natural and necessary, responsibility for others, and at least some degree of communitarianism.[19] It can also help move us from predominately law-based practice standards that are an integral part of the market, to a much greater role for ethics and ethical behavior in the practice of medicine.

CONCLUSION

The challenge to recreate a health care system that provides affordable high quality health care for all remains; and we will not face, let alone meet, this challenge if we continue to rely on visions of health care mediated by the military and market metaphors. Language powerfully affects how we think and is infectious: as William S. Burroughs has aptly put it, "language is a virus." We need a new vision of health care, and the ecology metaphor provides one that can directly address the major problems with our current culture, as well as the "deep" issues in health care. We need a metaphor that puts quality over quantity of life, and privileges ethics over legal considerations; we need a new metaphorical construct that can in turn lead society to think and act about health care in a new way. Adoption of the ecological metaphor could also help us confront what Vaclav Havel has called the end of the modern age, and move us to something new; a state of human affairs that values universal human rights, but also has space for an appreciation of "the miracle of being the miracle of the universe, the miracle of nature, the miracle of our own existence."[20]

REFERENCES

1. Lakoff G., Johnson M. Metaphors we live by. Chicago: University of Chicago Press, 1980.
2. Childress J. Who should decide? Paternalism in health care. New York: Oxford University Press, 1982: 7.
3. Sontag S. Illness as metaphor and AIDS and its metaphors, New York: Doubleday, 1990.
4. Fussell P. The great war and modern memory, New York: Oxford U. Press, 1975.
5. Keegan J. A history of warfare, New York: Vintage Books, 1994: 56–7.
6. Beisecker AE, Beisecker TD. Using metaphors to characterize doctor-patient relationships: paternalism versus consumerism. Health Communication 1993; 5:41–58.
7. Eckholm E. While congress remains silent, health care transforms itself, New York Times, Dec. 18, 1994: 1, 34 (quoting Uwe Reinhardt).

8. Relman AS. Shattack lecture: the health care industry: where is it taking us? N Engl J Med 1991: 854–859.

9. Relman AS. What market values are doing to medicine. Atlantic Monthly, March 1992: 99–106.

10. Bill and Hill , auditions for "Americas' funniest health videos", Boston Globe, March 27, 1994: 70.

11. Horwitz WA. Characteristics of environmental ethics: environmental activists' accounts. Ethics & Behavior 1994; 4:345–67.

12. Thomas L. The Lives of a cell. New York: Viking, 1974.

13. Potter, VR. Bioethics: Bridge to the future. Englewood Cliffs NJ: Prentice - Hall, 1971.

14. Sessions G. Ed. Deep ecology for the twenty-first century. Boston: Shambhala, 1995.

15. Gaylin W. Faulty diagnosis: why Clinton's health-care plan won't cure what ails us. Harper's , Oct., 1993, 57–62.

16. Editorial, Population health looking upstream. Lancet 1994; 343–429–30.

17. McKinlay JB. A case for refocusing upstream: the political economy of illness. Proceedings of American Heart Association Conferences on Applying Behavioral Science to Cardiovascular Risk. Seattle: American Health Association, 1974.

18. Dubos R. Mirage of health. New York: Harper, 1959: 233.

19. Friedman E. An ethic for all of us. Healthcare Forum J. March, 1991: 11–12.

20. Havel V. The new measure of man, New York Times. July 8, 1994: A27.

6

USES OF INFORMATION ABOUT HEALTH-RELATED QUALITY OF LIFE IN PATIENTS WITH AIDS AND CANCER

Paul D. Cleary

Department Health Care Policy
Harvard Medical School
Boston, Massachusetts

INTRODUCTION

The term "health-related quality of life" (HRQL) generally refers to aspects of people's lives that are important to them and that are directly related to, or affected by, their health or medical treatment (1–5). HRQL is related to the more general concept of "quality of life", but is less inclusive (6–9). Thus, when we talk about measuring quality of life in medical studies, we usually are referring to factors that can be directly affected by the way care is provided.

Most conceptualizations of HRQL include the dimensions of symptoms, physical functioning, social functioning, role functioning, mental health, disability, and general health perceptions, (2,10,11) with important concepts such as vitality (energy/fatigue), pain and cognitive functioning subsumed under these broader categories. (2,12).

Frequently, in studies of persons with AIDS and cancer, clinical treatments are expected to affect these aspects of HRQL. Those concepts are related in very complicated ways to physiological determinants of health and to medical treatments. Because of these complicated relationships, it is important to have a conceptual model to select the most appropriate measures of HRQL and to guide analyses of the impact of different medical treatments or interventions. However, there has been relatively little work to date that either explicitly conceptualizes the relationships of clinical variables to measures of HRQL or attempts to determine the intervening variables that mediate these effects (1,13–17). Wilson and Cleary (18) have developed a taxonomy of patient outcomes, that (a) categorizes measures of patient outcome according to the underlying health concepts they represent, and (b) proposes specific causal relationships between different health concepts, thereby integrating the two models of health described above.

In Wilson's model, measures of health are thought of as existing on a continuum of increasing biologic, social and psychologic complexity. At one end of the continuum are biologic measures, and at the other are more complex and integrated measures such as

Cancer, AIDS, and Quality of Life, edited by Levy *et al.*
Plenum Press, New York, 1997

physical functioning and general health perceptions. These relationships, as we conceptualize them, are displayed schematically in Figure 1. The arrows in Figure 1 do not imply that there are not reciprocal relationships. Neither does the absence of arrows between non-adjacent levels imply that there are not such relationships. The main purpose of the Figure is to distinguish among conceptually distinct measures of HRQL and to make explicit what we think are the dominant causal associations.

MEASUREMENT APPROACHES

There are several general measurement approaches to assessing HRQL. These include using: (a) Generic single measures, (b) Generic batteries, (c) Condition specific single scales, and (d) Condition specific batteries. Generic single measures, such as the QWB are useful for comparison across populations and are easy to summarize and use. However, they may obscure important differences in components, may be insensitive to condition-specific problems, and may be difficult to interpret clinically. Generic batteries, such as the SIP, SF-36, and EuroQol are useful for comparisons across populations, but may be insensitive to condition-specific problems. Condition specific single scales, such as the CARES and BCQ assess issues of particular salience to target populations and are easy to summarize and use, but they may obscure important differences in components and may be difficult to interpret clinically. Condition-specific batteries, such as the EORTC assess issues of particular salience to target populations but probably not optimal for comparing certain populations.

HRQL ASSESSMENT IN PERSONS WITH AIDS

We developed and used a new quality of life measure for persons with HIV infection and used it in face-to-face interviews with 189 AIDS patients in the Boston area. Follow-

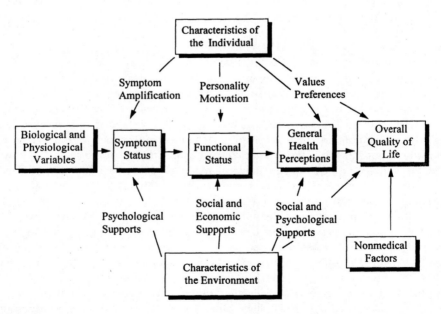

Figure 1. Relationships among measures of patient outcome in a health-related quality of life model.

ing the model developed by Wilson and Cleary, we think of symptoms as the most specific patient reported measures of health status. Measurements that are less specific but assess a broader range of consequences of illness include those of disability and functional status. The least specific and most comprehensive measures of health status are patients' global evaluations. In this study we grouped our measures in this way and we assessed: (a) which symptoms are most predictive of functional impairment and (b) which symptoms and which aspects of functional impairment best predict patients' overall perception of their health and their life satisfaction.

METHODS

We conducted a study at three sites: an academic group practice based at a private teaching hospital; a specialized ambulatory care clinic at a public teaching hospital; and a health maintenance organization. Patients were eligible for this study if they were diagnosed with AIDS and were current patients at one of the three study sites.

There were 293 eligible patients during the study period. Thirty-three patients died before they could be contacted. We successfully interviewed 189 patients, representing 65 percent of eligible patients. Respondents were not significantly different from the total eligible population with respect to age, gender, risk group, or race/ethnicity (19).

Most study participants were male, under the age of 35, white, and well educated. About 70 percent of the sample were men who said they considered themselves gay or bisexual. About seven percent of the sample were women and a quarter of all respondents said they had used illegal intravenous drugs. We have described the rationale and methods for the study and subject characteristics in detail elsewhere (19,20).

MEASURES

To assess HRQL, we developed a comprehensive set of subscales for assessing the symptoms and functioning of persons with HIV infection that includes HIV-specific measures of symptoms. The interview included: measures of life satisfaction (6); three items asking patients to rate their health at its best and worst during the preceding four months and how they felt, on average, during the previous month and on the day of the interview (on a scale ranging from 0 to 100); measures of basic and intermediate activities of daily living (e.g., "During the past month, about how many days did the way you felt make you *unable* to walk one block or climb one flight of stairs?) (4,11,21); emotional well-being (e.g., "How much of the time during the past month have you felt so down in the dumps that nothing could cheer you up?) (4,11,22); fatigue (e.g., "How much of the time during the past month did you feel worn out?") (23); disability (24); pain ("How much of the time during the past month have you been in extreme pain?"); and several neuropsychological tests to assess cognitive deficits (25). As part of the interview, we also asked respondents two questions about their memory from the Memory Assessment Clinic Self-Rating Scale (e.g., "In the last month, compared to the best your memory has ever been, how would you describe the speed with witch you remember things?") (26). These items were the best predictors of clinical assessments of HIV related cognitive deficits in a study of 129 patients evaluated for AIDS dementia complex.

We also asked respondents how much of the time in the previous month they had experienced each of 18 symptoms. To develop the list, we first compiled items from several unpublished AIDS symptom inventories. We then revised this list, based on advice from a panel of clinical consultants, to include symptoms thought to be especially important for HIV-infected persons. The final scale included seven symptoms related to neurological complications of HIV infection, three sleep-related symptoms, three fever-related symptoms, and five other general symptoms.

SUMMARY OF RESULTS

We have described the results from this study in more detail elsewhere (20), but several findings illustrate the importance of differentiating among HRQL measures. For example, although some HRQL scales combine symptom and functioning measures, our results emphasize the importance of separating them when developing theoretical and statistical models.

Our first step in developing such a model was to examine the extent to which symptoms predicted limitations in functioning. One finding is that every symptom measure was more strongly correlated with limitations in intermediate activities of daily living (IADL) than with basic activities of daily living (BADL). The standard deviation of the IADL scores is higher than for the BADL score, so we do not think this is an artifact of the variances of the scales. We think it is likely that symptoms have little effect on one's ability to carry out basic activities, but are related to more complex functions.

A second important finding was that the patterns of associations were not consistent with some of our clinical predictions. For example, we thought that specific symptoms such as fever, nausea, and diarrhea would be better predictors than more diffuse symptoms, such as fatigue. Surprisingly, diarrhea and fever had among the lowest correlations with IADL scores and fatigue had one of the highest correlations with the IADL score. The variable with the highest correlation with the IADL score was a summary score that represented the sum of the individual physical symptom scores.

In a regression model, the only symptom measure that was an independent predictor of problems with basic ADLs was the physical symptom score. The physical symptom score and reported fatigue were independent predictors of both limitations in intermediate ADLs and disability days.

PREDICTORS OF SUMMARY VARIABLES

Another implication of the model described above is that it is important to distinguish overall health perception from symptom and functioning measures. Although most HRQL scales include both, little attention generally is given to the associations between these different levels of measurement. Analyzing the data in this way yields several unanticipated findings and raises important theoretical questions. For example, our initial hypothesis was that health perceptions would be influenced most by variables most proximate in our model, such as the limitations in IADL.

It is noteworthy that, the strongest correlate was the measure of fatigue. The next strongest correlates were limitations in IADLs and the summary physical symptom score. The weakest correlates were reported sleep problems, diarrhea, and limitations in basic ADLs. As expected, the symptom and functioning measures had weaker correlations with the rating of life satisfaction than with the rating of physical health.

This is consistent with our assumption that many factors besides symptoms and functional status influence life satisfaction. The strongest correlates of life satisfaction were fatigue and the physical symptom score. The other symptom and functioning measures were moderately correlated with life satisfaction.

When the rating of average health in the previous month was regressed on the symptom and functioning measures, the significant predictors were bed disability days, fatigue, and the physical symptom score. The significant predictors of the mental health score were the intermediate ADL score, the measure of fatigue, and the physical symptom score.

A linear regression in which life satisfaction was a dependent variable showed that the summary health rating and the mental health score explained 27 percent of the variance in life satisfaction and that none of the other symptom or functioning measures were significant predictors of life satisfaction.

HRQL ASSESSMENT IN PERSONS WITH PROSTATE CANCER

We recently developed a set of HRQL measures to include in a multicenter randomized trial to compare the effects of different treatments on in-patients with advanced prostate cancer (27). A total of 487 patients were enrolled in Austria, Denmark, Holland, Norway, Sweden, and the United Kingdom. In that study, we assessed several dimensions of HRQL: symptoms, pain, physical functioning, social functioning, sexual interest, sexual functioning, emotional well-being, memory problems, disability, and perceived global health. Among the issues examined in this study were the reliability and validity of different HRQL scales after translation into different languages.

To compare the construct validity of the scales in the different countries, we calculated the Pearson product-moment correlation between each of the scales and patients' global health assessment. These data are presented in Table 1.

These data suggest that although some of the scales, such as those measuring fatigue, pain, and functioning are related to general health perceptions across the different countries in the trial, there were substantial differences in the correlations between general health perceptions and the measures of sexual functioning. These results emphasize both the validity of certain measures in this type of study and the potential difficulties of using

Table 1. International study of patients with advanced prostate cancer correlations between global health perceptions and other HRQL measures

MEASURE	COUNTRY					
	AUSTRIA	DENMARK	HOLLAND	NORWAY	SWEDEN	UK
PAIN	-0.56	-0.54	-0.49	-0.51	-0.41	-0.44
FATIGUE	-0.83	0.72	0.78	0.77	0.74	0.74
SEXUAL INTEREST	0.30	0.20	0.32	0.11	0.01	0.06
SEXUAL FUNCTIONING	--	0.27	--	-0.37	-0.28	0.01

measures of sensitive or subjective topics in different cultures, with instruments that have been translated into different languages.

POTENTIAL USES OF HRQL INFORMATION IN CLINICAL ENCOUNTERS, CLINICAL TRIALS, AND MAKING DECISIONS ABOUT RESOURCE

As we have indicated above, there are numerous approaches to assessing health-related quality of life and literally hundreds of reliable, valid, and easily administered scales for assessing both health status and patients' preferences for different states of health. There is a great deal of confusion and disagreement, however, over definitions of terms in this area. There also is disagreement over how health status and patient preferences should be measured and how such information can best be used in different situations. Tsevat and colleagues (28) have developed a taxonomy of quality of life measures, classifying them by what they measure, how they measure it, and how they are scored. They also discuss how quality of life information might best be collected and used in each of three settings: 1) the clinical encounter, 2) clinical trials, and 3) health policy. I summarize some of the main points from that paper below.

THE CLINICAL ENCOUNTER

In some clinical situations, one treatment is so obviously preferable to the alternatives that quality of life data are not helpful for guiding clinical decisions. In many clinical situations, though, there are several possible treatments for which mortality is comparable, for which death is not a likely outcome, or for which potential changes in survival must be balanced against potential changes in quality of life. In such cases, the relevant information might include the effect of the therapy on quality of life. In the following sections, we discuss several common clinical situations that help elucidate the types of information that would most facilitate clinical decision making.

The Competent, Willing Decision Maker

To make an informed choice, a patient who is competent and wishes to be involved in decision making should have complete data on the expected outcomes of each possible treatment strategy (29). These data should include not only physiologic outcomes such as survival but also health status information.

If alternative treatments offer similar life expectancy and differ only with respect to their impact on certain aspects of health then the patient will need data about the effects of each treatment on health status. For example, one cancer treatment may involve more short-term toxicity but result in better long-term functional status than another, or may result in less pain but also in less mobility than another. With information about the likelihood of different outcomes, the patient can decide, using his or her own values, which set of outcomes he or she prefers.

The Reluctant Decision Maker

Patients may not always be able to use health status data to make decisions. They may be too distressed to evaluate clinical alternatives, may be overwhelmed by the complexity of the task, may not know what they value or how to compare values, or may simply prefer to defer the decision (29,30). To the extent that the decision involves a trade-off of one desirable outcome for another or one undesirable outcome for another, the relative importance of those outcomes should be evaluated. If patients can provide any information at all about how they value those outcomes, then those preferences should be used.

The Patient Who Cannot Participate in Decision Making

If the patient cannot supply any information about his or her values then someone else must make the decision. In practice, most physicians would rely on mortality data in recommending a course of action. To the extent that physicians consider information on other outcomes, they probably would apply their own values or the values of other health care professionals to those outcomes. Because those values and preferences are often incongruent with those of patients (31–33), perhaps a preferable alternative would be to use the values of previous similar patients, if such data are available. Those preferences could have been obtained formally or indirectly by observing choices made by patients who had been fully informed of the relevant survival and health status data.

CLINICAL TRIALS

Increasingly, clinicians, researchers, and policy makers agree that quality of life information is usually useful and often essential in evaluating the results of clinical trials, especially when the interventions being evaluated have a comparable impact on survival. Also, the evaluation of interventions sometimes involves trade-offs between survival and quality of life or between one aspect of quality of life and another. Preference assessments can be used to calculate and compare quality-adjusted survival in trials of interventions that improve some outcomes and worsen others or trials that involve trade-offs between survival and quality of life. As an example, Coates and co-workers (34) studied the impact on survival and quality of life of two strategies for treating women with metastatic breast cancer: continuous vs. intermittent chemotherapy. They found that survival in the two arms was not significantly different, but that patients in the continuous treatment group scored higher on serial health status measures of overall quality of life and on all attribute-specific measures except nausea. The authors concluded that continuous chemotherapy was a better strategy. Had they found that patients on continuous therapy lived slightly longer but experienced worse quality of life than patients on intermittent therapy, or that survival was equivalent but patients in the continuous therapy arm reported more nausea, depression, and anxiety but better functional status, then identifying the "better" strategy would have been problematic.

RESOURCE ALLOCATION

Using health status and value information to develop measures of the relative value of different treatments is complicated and the data necessary for such calculations often are not available. Furthermore, considerations such as the concerns of particularly needy population subgroups or inclinations to fund heroic life-saving procedures ("rule of rescue") may play as great a role as information about the impact of quality of life when making allocation decisions (35,36). Nevertheless, information about the impact of treatments on health status and the value of those outcomes to the persons affected can help make explicit the types of trade-offs that usually are implicit in allocation decisions.

If one accepts the premise that program comparison should be based on the impact of treatments on different outcomes and that values can be used to combine information on different outcomes, the question becomes whose values should be used. Different groups do not assign the same values to health states.

One could argue that when society is paying for medical care or when treatment has an impact on society (e.g., treatment of infectious diseases), society should determine the values. Alternatively, healthy members of society may not know what it is like to have a particular illness or treatment.

In spite of these complexities, routinely collecting data on both the health status outcomes of different medical treatments and patients' preferences for different health states would focus attention on these issues and would help policy makers explicate the rationale behind policies affecting the allocation of scarce resources.

CONCLUSION

Patients, clinicians, researchers, policy makers, the courts, and pharmaceutical companies have come to recognize the significance of quality of life and patient preferences. The federal government, through the Agency for Health Care Policy and Research, is particularly interested in using such outcomes to evaluate the effectiveness of different types of medical and surgical treatment. In spite of this increased interest and the plethora of instruments, much confusion remains. If this confusion continues, it is likely that decision makers will either neglect this information altogether or measure and collect it without adequately considering its proper use and interpretation.

A major step in reducing confusion and facilitating the use of information about health status and preferences is to clarify the situations in which the information should be used. The information needed for different types of decisions may be quite different. In some situations, such as decision making involving the competent, willing patient, information about the changes in health that are likely to result from treatment may be adequate and probably are the most appropriate information to provide. For other patients and for resource allocation, information about both health status and health values are desirable. Clinical trials can provide a rich source of both health status and preference data, useful for interpretation of the trials themselves and for the aforementioned decision making paradigms.

Health-related quality of life (HRQL) is increasingly used as an outcome in clinical trials, effectiveness research, and research on quality of care involving persons with AIDS and cancer. Factors which have facilitated this increased usage include the accumulating evidence that measures of HRQL are "valid" and "reliable," (37) the publication of clinical trials showing that these outcome measures are responsive to important clinical changes (38–41), and the successful development and testing of shorter instruments that are easier to understand and administer (42–48). These measures are useful and important supplements to traditional physiologic or biologic measures of health status and, if used more systematically, could improve clinical decision making, help interpret better the results of selected clinical trails, and help explicate some of the assumptions underlying resource allocation decisions.

REFERENCES

1. Patrick DL, Bergner M. Measurement of health status in the 1990's. Ann Rev Public Health. 1990;11:165–183.
2. Ware JE. Standards for validating health measures: Definition and content. J Chronic Dis. 1987;40:473–480.
3. Bergner M. Quality of care, health status, and clinical research. Med Care. 1989;27:S148-S156.
4. Cleary PD, Greenfield S, McNeil BJ. Assessing quality of life after surgery. Controlled Clin Trials. 1991;12:189S-203S.
5. Stewart AL. The medical outcomes study framework of health indicators. In: Stewart AL, Ware JE Jr. (Ed.). Measuring functioning and well-being. The medical outcomes study approach. Durham: Duke University Press, 1992:12–24.
6. Andrews FM, Withey SB. Social indicators of well-being: Americans' perceptions of life quality. New York: Plenum, 1976.
7. Burt RS, Wiley JA, Minor MJ, Murray JR. Structure of well-being form, content, and stability over time. Sociol Meth Res. 1978;6:365–407.
8. Flanagan JC. A research approach to improving our quality of life. Am Psychologist. 1978;33:138–147.
9. Patrick DL, Erickson P. Assessing health-related quality of life for clinical decision making. In: Walker Sr, Rosser RM (Ed.). Quality of Life: Assessment and Application. Lancaster, England: MTP Press Ltd., 1988:9.
10. Ware JE, Brook RH, Davies AR, Lohr KN. Choosing measures of health status for individuals in general populations. Am J Public Health. 1981;71:620–625.
11. Jette AM, Davies AR, Cleary PD, Calkins DR, Rubenstein LV, Fink A, Kosecoff J, Young RT, Brook RH, Delbanco TL. The functional status questionnaire: Its reliability and validity when used in primary care. J Gen Intern Med. 1986;1:143–149.
12. Fries JF. The hierarchy of quality-of-life assessment, the Health Assessment Questionnaire (HAQ), and issues mandating development of a toxicity index. Controlled Clin Trials. 1991;12:106S-117S.
13. Bergner M. Measurement of health status. Med Care. 1985;23:696–704.
14. Nagi S. Some conceptual issues in disability and rehabilitation. In: M.B. Sussman (Ed.). Sociology and Rehabilitation. Washing. D.C.:Am Sociological Assoc., 1965.
15. Read JL, Quinn RJ, Hoefer MA. Measuring overall health: An evaluation of three important approaches. J Chron Dis. 1987;40:7S-21S.
16. Verbrugge LM. Physical and social disability in adults. In: H Hibbard, PA Nutting, and ML Grady (Ed.). Primary Care Research: Theory and Methods. U.S. Dept. of Health and Human Services, 1991:31–53.
17. Johnson RJ, Wolinsky FD. The structure of health status among older adults: disease, disability, functional limitation, and perceived health. J Hlth Soc Beh. 1993;34:105–121.
18. Wilson IB, Cleary PD. Linking clinical variables with health-related quality of life: A causal model of patient outcomes. JAMA. 1995;273:59–65.
19. Fowler FJ Jr., Massagli MP, Weissman J, Seage GR, Cleary PD, Epstein A. Some methodological lessons for surveys of persons with AIDS. Med Care. 1992;30:1059–1066.
20. Cleary PD, Fowler FJ Jr, Weissman J, Massagli MP, Wilson I, Seage GR, Gatsonis C, Epstein A. Health-related quality of life in persons with AIDS. Med Care. 1993;31:569–580.
21. Jette AM, Cleary, PD. Functional disability assessment. Phys Ther. 1987;67:1854–1859.
22. Cleary PD, Greenfield S, Mulley AG, et al. Variations in length of stay and outcomes for six medical and surgical conditions in Massachusetts and California. JAMA. 1991;266:73–79.
23. Stewart AL, Hays RD, Ware JE Jr. The MOS short-form General Health Survey: Reliability and validity in a patient population. Med Care. 1988;26:724–735.
24. National Center for Health Statistics. National Health Interview Survey, 1986: Interviewer's manual, HIS-100. Hyattsville, MD: National Center for Health Statistics, 1987.
25. Price RW, Brew B, Sidtis J, Rosenblum M, Scheck AC, Cleary P. The brain in AIDS: Central nervous system HIV-1 infection and AIDS dementia complex. Science. 1988;239:586–592.
26. Winterling D, Crook T, Salama M, Gobert J. A self-rating scale for assessing memory loss. Bethesda, MD: Memory Assessment Clinics Inc., 1986:482–487.
27. Cleary PD, Morrissey G, Oster G. Health-related quality of life in patients with advanced prostate cancer: A multinational perspective. Quality of Life Research. 1995; 4:207–20.
28. Tsevat J, Weeks JC, Guadagnoli E, Tosteson ANA, Mangione CM, Pliskin JS, Weinstein MC, Cleary PD. Using health-related quality of life information: clinical encounters, clinical trials, and health policy. J Gen Intern Med. 1994;9:576–581.

29. Emanuel EJ, Emanuel LL. Four models of the physician-patient relationship. JAMA. 1992;267:2221–2226.
30. Fischhoff, B. Value elicitation: Is there anything in there? Am Psychologist. 1991;46:835–847.
31. Tsevat J, Cook EF, Phillips RS, et al. How do utilities of seriously ill patients compare with those of their nurses and health care proxies? (abstract). Clin Res. 1991;40:568A.
32. Phillips RS, Teno J, Wenger N, et al. Physicians' preferences for cardiopulmonary resuscitation: accuracy and correlates of discordance (abstract). Clin Res. 1992;40:617A.
33. Wenger NS, Oye RK, Teno JM, et al. Physicians often do not know patients' goals for care: factors associated with misunderstanding (abstract). Clin Res. 1992;40:620A.
34. Coates A, Gebski V, Bishop JF, et. al. Improving the quality of life during chemotherapy for advanced breast cancer. N Engl J Med. 1987;317:1490–1495.
35. Hadorn DC. Setting health care priorities in Oregon: cost-effectiveness meets the rule of rescue. JAMA. 1991;265:2218–2225.
36. Eddy DM. Oregon's methods: did cost-effectiveness analysis fail? JAMA. 1991;266:2135–2141.
37. McDowell I, Newell C. Measuring Health: A Guide to Rating Scales and Questionnaires. New York: Oxford University Press, 1987.
38. Croog SH, Levine S, Testa MA, Brown B, Bulpitt CJ, Jenkins CD, Klerman GL, Williams GH. The effects of antihypertensive therapy on the quality of life. N Engl J Med. 1986;314:1657–1664.
39. Bombardier C, Ware J, Russell IJ, Larson M, Chalmers A, Read JL, and the Auranofin Cooperating Group. Auranofin therapy and quality of life in patients with rheumatoid arthritis. Am J Med. 1986;81:565–578.
40. Canadian Erythropoietin Study Group. Association between recombinant human erythropoietin and quality of life and exercise capacity of patients receiving haemodialysis. Br Med J. 1990;300:573–578.
41. Cleary PD, Epstein AM, Oster G, Morrissey GS, Stason WB, Debussey S, Plachetka J, Zimmerman M. Health-related quality of life among patients undergoing percutaneous transluminal coronary angioplasty. Med Care. 1991;29:939–950.
42. Parkerson GR, Broadhead WE. Tse CJ. The Duke health profile. A 17-item measure of health and dysfunction. Med Care. 1990;28:1056–1072.
43. Hunt SM, McEwen J, McKenna SP. Measuring health status: a new tool for clinicians and epidemiologists. J Roy Coll Gen Pract. 1985;35:185–188.
44. Nelson EC, Wasson JH, Krik JW. Assessment of function in routine clinical practice: Description of the COOP Chart method and preliminary findings. J Chronic Dis. 1987;40 (suppl 1):55S-63S.
45. McHorney CA, Ware JE, Rogers W, Raczek AE, Lu JFR. The validity and relative precision of MOS short- and long- form health status scales and Dartmouth COOP charts. Med Care. 1992;30:MS253-MS265.
46. Ware JE, Sherbourne CD. The MOS 36-item short-form health survey (SF-36) 1. conceptual framework and item selection. Med Care. 1992;30:473–483.
47. McHorney CA, Ware JE Jr., Raczek AE. The MOS 36-item short-form health survey (SF-36): II. Psychometric and clinical tests of validity in measuring physical and mental health conditions. Med Care. 1993;31:247–263.
48. McHorney CA, Ware JE, Lu JFR, Sherbourne CD. The MOS short-form health survey (SF-36): III. Tests of data quality, scaling assumptions, and reliability across diverse patient groups. Med Care. 1994;32:40–66.

7

IMPROVING THE QUALITY OF LIFE OF CANCER PATIENTS

Peter Maguire

Christie Hospital NHS Trust
Stanley House, Wilmslow Road
M20 4BX Withington
Manchester, United Kingdom

INTRODUCTION

Recent research found that 33% of cancer patients still develop anxiety and depression as a result of their diagnosis and treatment [1]. This anxiety and depression seriously impairs the quality of patients' lives. It causes much personal suffering, interferes with their day to day functioning, delays return to work, affects their personal relationships and decision making. So, it is important to find ways of preventing the development of these affective disorders.

IMPROVING INFORMATION GIVING

A follow up study of breast cancer patients [2] found a strong relationship between the development of affective disorders and the information given to patients at the time of diagnosis. Patients who considered that the information they were given about diagnosis and treatment was adequate to their needs coped well psychologically. In contrast, those who felt they were given too much information or too little were more likely to develop an affective disorder. The challenge, therefore, for the health professional is to learn how to tailor information to meet the needs of each individual rather than taking refuge in rules about telling or not telling.

Most patients presenting with symptoms suggestive of a cancer diagnosis have realised already that the diagnosis is probable. If the clinician checks, therefore, their perception of what might be wrong it will become evident that they have considered that it could be cancer. Thus, if the clinician is prepared to ask "What have you made of these symptoms"? or "What do you think all this might be due to"? 80% of patients will reply that they think it could be cancer. The clinician's task is then to indicate that they are correct and so confirm the bad news.

Cancer, AIDS, and Quality of Life, edited by Levy *et al.*
Plenum Press, New York, 1997

In those 20% of patients who have no idea or only a slight suspicion that they have cancer it is important to check how much they want to know by giving the information in a series of steps. Thus, the clinician should start with giving a warning shot by saying, for example, I am afraid the condition looks serious. The patient who wants to know more will ask "What do you mean serious"? The patient who does not want more information will say 'I don't want to know the details, just tell me what you are going to be able to do".

When patients indicate they want to know in what way the condition is serious a further euphemism can be used like 'It looks as though you have a tumour'. Patients can again respond and ask what the clinician means by "tumour" or indicate that they do not wish to proceed along the truth telling pathway. Finally, the clinician can respond to the question "What do you mean tumour" by saying that it is a cancer.

ELICITING PATIENTS' CONCERNS

One of the best predictors of psychological adjustment after a cancer diagnosis is the extent to which patients' concerns have been disclosed and resolved. Patients who have more undisclosed concerns and concerns of greater severity are more likely to develop a major depressive illness or generalised anxiety disorder [1]. However, in practice the majority of patients' concerns remain undisclosed. There is a marked selectivity in patients' disclosure. They prefer to offer concerns about physical aspects of their illness and treatment rather than psychological and social concerns [3].

Certain interviewing skills improve markedly the chances of patients disclosing their concerns thus allowing clinicians to try to help resolve them.

When bad news has been confirmed or broken it is important to acknowledge patients' distress by saying "I can see this has been very upsetting for you" and then ask what concerns the patient has about the situation. It is important to follow up and clarify any resulting cues, for example, worries about pain, survival and the effect on the family. Having elicited their main concerns it is important to ask patients to put these in priority order in case there is not sufficient time to deal with all of them within the consultation. Patients need to know their concerns have been elicited and acknowledged and that something will be done about them when possible.

CONCLUSION

By tailoring information to the needs of patients, by eliciting their distress and the concerns that are causing that distress before attempting to give advice and information the development of affective disorders should be considerably reduced and quality of their lives improved.

HINDERING DISCLOSURE

Certain interviewing behaviours hinder disclosure and, therefore, their use leads to an impaired quality of life. Moving into advice and information mode before the patients concerns have been elicited is especially inhibitory. It is common for clinicians at the time of breaking bad news to respond immediately to patients' distress by talking about how they plan to erradicate or control the cancer and discuss the treatments that might be involved. If this is done the patient remains preoccupied with their concerns while they are being given key information. Consequently, they remember little of the positive information and recall selectively negative statements like "We are going to give you radiotherapy because there may be some residual cancer cells".

TRAINING OF HEALTH PROFESSIONALS

Unfortunately, health professionals use as many if not more behaviours that inhibit patient disclosure of concerns than behaviours that promote it. Training methods have been developed which help them acquire the positive skills and relinquish the inhibitory ones [4]. This should markedly help improve patients quality of life.

REFERENCES

1. Parle M, Jones B, Maguire P. Maladaptive coping and affective disorders in cancer patients. Psychological Medicine, 26, In Press.
2. Fallowfield LJ, Hall A, Maguire GP, Baum M. (1990) Psychological outcomes of different treatment policies in women with early breast cancer outside a clinical trial. BMJ, 301: 575–580.
3. Heaven CM, Maguire P. (1996) Training hospice nurses to elicit patients' concerns. J of Adv Nursing, 23: 280–286.
4. Maguire P. (19/95) Psychosocial interventions to reduce affective disorders in cancer patients: Research Priorities. Psycho-Oncology, 4: 113–119.

8

HOW DOES THE COST OF CARE INFLUENCE THE EFFECTIVENESS OF HEALTH CARE DELIVERY?

Joan Rovira and Patricia Alegre

Soikos SE
c/Sardenya 229 237 64
08013
Barcelona, España

INTRODUCTORY REMARKS

This paper addresses the issue of how economists -or rather, how economic analysis- approaches the issue of quality of life in relation to health care in general and, more specifically, in relation to the efficiency of the treatment of cancer and AIDS. Economic analysis is concerned with human wellbeing and how this is affected by the allocation of limited resources. Economic analysis must address issues of how to allocate limited budgets among treatments for patients whose needs are practically unlimited. We can state that there is a need of health care if there is an effective treatment for a given condition, i.e., if an individual's health status can be improved by providing him or her a certain type and amount of health care.

The economic criterion of efficiency can be interpreted as the requirement that resources are allocated so as to maximise health or wellbeing. According to the famous WHO definition, health is identified with wellbeing; however, for most people the concept of wellbeing is a broader one. Smoking or fast driving does apparently contribute to the wellbeing of some individuals, although few would state that it contributes to their health. These issues are likely to prove very important in the case of irreversible diseases, specially at their terminal stages, when no cure can be expected and increased survival may imply additional years in highly deteriorated and painful living conditions, as it is often the case of AIDS and cancer patients.

Quality of life is a concept with different meanings and contents, which vary according to the purpose and to the disciplinary context in which it is used. There is no point in trying to find a single right definition; different definitions may be appropriate for different purposes. Clinical and psychometric researchers usually conceptualize health related quality of life (HRQL) as a multiattribute function of health status, consisting of a set of dimensions each of which can be assigned a score. A combination of these scores repre-

Cancer, AIDS, and Quality of Life, edited by Levy *et al.*
Plenum Press, New York, 1997

sents the HRQL of a given health state. Sometimes all of these scores can be combined into a single general score.

The comparison of the output of various treatments or interventions - which is a condition for comparing efficiency - requires the output to be measured in the same unit. Years of life gained sometimes has been used as such a unit. However, this approach is only valid for comparing treatments that increase survival and when that survival is assumed to be of similar quality or value for the individuals. As this is usually not the case, economists developed the concept of quality adjusted life year (QALY). The QALY approach assumes that health has two basic dimensions: length of life and quality of life. Quality of life is defined as the value associated to a given health state that allows years of life to be expressed in a single unit. Quality of life is usually a value between one - the quality of life of perfect health - and zero - the quality of life of the worst possible state, which is often identified with death. For instance, an additional survival of 8 years which has an associated quality of life of 0.25 is equivalent to two years in full health or to four years in a state with a 0.5 value: $8 \times 0.25 = 2 \times 1 = 4 \times 0.5 = 2$ QALYs.

The concept of the Q-TWIST, (Quality of life related to Time Without Symptoms and Toxicity) derived from the QALY unit and has been specifically used in the economic analysis of cancer and AIDS treatments. Its advantage is to measure the variations in quality of life between treatments or interventions when a significant increase in survival has not been proved.

The effects of an intervention are expressed in an economic evaluation in terms of its cost per QALY gained (net increase in resource use divided by net increase in QALYs). If one wants to maximize QALYs gained subject to a resource constraint, interventions should be implemented according to the value of the cost per QALY or the cost-utility ratio. Those interventions with the lowest ratio should be given priority. Ideally, all available interventions should be ordered according to the cost-utility ratio and resources should be sequentially allocated to the interventions until all available resources have been exhausted.

ECONOMIC EVALUATION IN CANCER AND AIDS TREATMENTS

Our purpose is to illustrate by examples different types of economic evaluation in cancer and AIDS treatments. They are based on units like:

- cost/year of life gained
- cost/QALY (Quality Adjusted Life Year)
- cost/Q-TWIST (Quality of life related to Time Without Symptoms and Toxicity)

A recent bibliography research showed that the incremental cost of an adjuvant chemotherapy after a surgery in the Dukes' C colonic carcinoma is 2.917 $/year of life saved, or 17.000$/QALY (1). The incremental cost of an autologous bone marrow transplantation versus a standard chemotherapy in the metastatic breast cancer is 115.800 $/year of life saved or 100.000$/QALY (2). These two treatments can define a scale within which different costs of therapies may be observed from standard to expensive high technology cancer interventions. The therapy with the lowest ratio could be the most efficient but it does not mean that is the society's preference because it does not integrate variations in patients' quality of life.

Thus, we can see in Table 1 that the scale is disorganised when we represent increasing treatment costs/QALY. The discord between the two treatments is shorter be-

Table 1. Cancer and AIDS treatments: Cost-utility ratios for economic evaluation

Treatment	Survival increase (months)	Quality of life (Quality adjusted months)	Incremental cost ($)	Incremental cost/QALY ($/QALY)	Cost/YOL ($/year of life saved)
Dukes' C colonic carcinoma (1): (1 247 patients)					
Adjuvant chemotherapy versus surgery alone	+ 28.8	+ 4.8	7,000	+ 17,500	+ 2,917
Early breast cancer for premenopausal women (3): (75,000 women)					
Estrogen dependant tumour:	NA[1]				
Tamoxifen (2-5 years) versus no treatment		from 3,49 to 5,17	2,500	from 4,330 to 11,440	NA
CMF (6 months) versus no treatment		from 4,09 to 5,82	6,000	from 9,230 to 11,370	
Tamoxifen + CMF versus CMF alone	NA	from 1,23 to 2,11	2,500	from 14,750 to 33,100	
Estrogen independant tumour:					
Tamoxifen (2-5 years) versus no treatment		from 0,17 to 0,40	2,500	from 57,800 to 214,000	NA
CMF (6 months) versus no treatment		from 9,20 to 10,7	6,000	from 4,890 to 4,970	
Tamoxifen + CMF versus CMF alone		from 0,20 to 0,39	2,500	from 80,700 to 186,200	
Metastatic breast cancer (2): (economic model)					
ABMT[2] versus standard chemotherapy	+ 6	+ 6,3	53,600	+ 96,600	+ 115,800
HIV patients with cough or dyspnea (13): (economic model)					
Beginning treatment with sputum analysis when CD4 < 200/mm^3	NA	+ 3,5	2,490	+ 34,174	NA

[1]Not available; autologous bone marrow transplantation. In the second example, treatments improve much more quality of life in premenopausal women with progressive disease in the lymphatic nodes (bad prognostic) than in women without that evolution. That can explain the lower cost/QALY ratios for the women with worst prognostic. Smith and Hillner, J. Clin. Oncol., 1993; 11:771-76

cause the autologous bone marrow transplantation provides a better quality adjusted months to patients. Therefore, the choice of a therapy based on an economic evaluation can be different from the previous approach.

Nevertheless, we must be careful when we compare cost/QALY ratios in different therapeutic areas for decision making. We have to make sure that the same point of view is adopted in the economic evaluations (society's or patients' point of view for instance) and that a QALY unit in one therapeutic area is equivalent to a QALY unit in another one. For example, can we say that oncologists and virologists value quality of life in cancer patients and in AIDS patients in an identical way? It is necessary to know this point if we want to compare costs/QALY for cancer and AIDS treatments.

Decision making based on cost/QALY ratios is easier when the QALYs of different treatments in a single therapeutic area are measured by the same sample of people (same point of view for each QALY).

Thus, we represented in Figure 1 the average cost/QALY related with the quality adjusted months for premenopausal women suffering from an early breast cancer with or without estrogen receptors (ER+ and ER- women) and treated by tamoxifen (anti-estrogenic drug) for two to five years or by CMF (Cyclophosphamide, Methotrexate, 5-Fluorouracil) for six months or both (3). For ER+ women, tamoxifen affords an average incremental 4,33 quality adjusted months compared with no treatment for 7.885 $/QALY (average incremental cost/QALY). CMF and tamoxifen +CMF increase quality of life respectively by 14% and 53% and cost/QALY by 31% and 334% .

For ER- women, tamoxifen versus no treatment improves slightly the quality adjusted months. The value of the average incremental quality adjusted months is 0,28. This corresponds to an average incremental cost/QALY of 135.900 $/QALY. The average incremental quality adjusted months of CMF and tamoxifen+CMF grows from 0,28 to 9,95 and 10,24 respectively. Compared with no treatment, their incremental costs/QALY are 4.930 and 138.380 $/QALY.

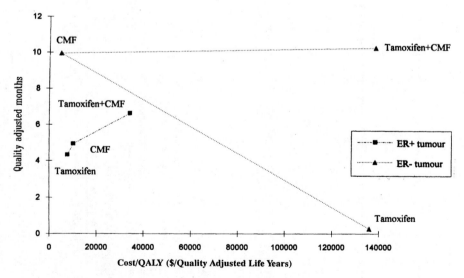

Figure 1. Quality of Life and cost of treatment in breast cancer patients.

Different parameters may influence the cost/QALY in cancer treatments like recurrence rate and expected life span of patients. A reduction in contralateral tumours would be beneficial and reduce the costs. However, an increased risk of secondary cancers like endometrial carcinoma when tamoxifen is used (4, 5) would reduce the number of QALYs gained and also add to the costs both in terms of treatment and follow up.

In Figure 1, it can be seen that tamoxifen in ER- women is inefficient because we can afford them treatments with an higher quality of life at a lower cost/QALY: CMF or tamoxifen+CMF. Tamoxifen+CMF presents a very high cost/QALY compared to CMF alone with a little increase in quality adjusted life. In the context of unlimited resources, the right choice for the ER- women's treatment would be tamoxifen+CMF. But, our economic context is not the same. We have got limited resources and the aim of the economist and the physician in health care is to allocate them optimally respecting medical ethics. Can we refuse to ER- women the tamoxifen+CMF treatment because it is too expensive? But, can the marginal costs be beared by the society? The same questions are asked concerning ER+women.

It is difficult to answer these questions while there is no general consensus on an upper limit of the cost therapy. According to Epstein in 1992 (6), 30.000 $/QALY could be an acceptable cut-off point for a patient. If we accept this figure, decision making based on a cost-utility analysis would be: CMF treatment for both ER- women and ER+women.

The characteristic of cancer and AIDS treatments is that until now they are symptomatic or palliative with a large toxicity and that in the majority of cases they have not proven a significant increase in overall survival. For this reason, the Q-TWIST model integrates three features for the comparison of treaments in terms of quality of life:

- Time without symptoms and toxicity (TWIST)
- Time with adverse events or toxicity (AE)
- Time of disease progression or relapse (PROG).

Q-TWIST, measured in months, is calculated as follows:

$$Q\text{-}TWIST = TWIST + U_{AE} \times AE + U_{PROG} \times PROG$$

U_{AE} and U_{PROG} are utility coefficients used to reflect the value of the state of health on a utility scale with reference points of 0 and 1: TWIST is assigned a weight of one and death a weight of zero.

If we postulated that $U_{AE} = U_{PROG} = 0,5$, six or seven cures of CMF after surgery improve quality of life compared to only one cure for pre- or postmenopausal women (7) (Table 2). In both groups, the chemotherapy increases TWIST but also AE. In addition, PROG is shorter. The incremental cost/Q-TWIST is 2.143 $/Q-TWIST for premenopausal women and 4.000 $/Q-TWIST for postmenopausal women.

Then, when an improvement in survival is not shown clearly in recurrent diseases, Q-TWIST is the better model to compare effects of drugs or interventions on quality of life. It can be applied with each patient's preferences. The choice of U_{AE} and U_{PROG} by the patient allows to adapt specifically the best treatment to her, respecting an acceptable cost for the society.

The Q-TWIST model has also been employed in measuring the pertinence of using AZT (zidovudine) in mildly symptomatic or asymptomatic HIV patients. The fact is that whether AZT improves survival is still controversial (8) (9). However, there is some evidences that AZT delays progression to ARC (AIDS Related Complex) or AIDS phases but

Table 2. Cancer and AIDS: Treatment costs and Q-TWIST model

Treatment	Overall survival (months)	Δ Twist (months)	Δ AE (months)	Δ Prog (months)	Δ Q-Twist (months)	Incremental Cost ($)	Incremental Cost/Δ Q-Twist ($/months)
CMF[1] for operable breast cancer in (7)(3):							
Premenopausal women	+ 2,6	+ 3,0	+ 5,1	- 5,5	+ 2,8	+ 6,000	+ 2,143
Postmenopausal women	+ 1,3	+ 1,8	+ 4,7	- 5,2	+ 1,5	+ 6,000	+ 4,000
(6 or 7 cures versus 1 cure of CMF in 1229 patients)							
AZT[2] in 711 mildly symptomatic HIV patients during 18 months (11) (14):							
1200 mg/day versus placebo	- 0,10	- 0,20	+ 1,10	- 1,00	- 0,15	+ 8,656	- 57,707
AZT in 1338 asymptomatic HIV patients during 18 months (13) (14):							
500 mg/day versus placebo	+ 0,03	- 0,08	+ 0,6	- 0,5	- 0,03	+ 3,979	- 132,633
1500 mg/day versus placebo	- 0,03	- 0,8	+ 1,2	- 0,3	- 0,35	+ 10,660	- 30,457
500 mg/day versus AZT 1,500 mg/day	+ 0,06	+ 0,8	- 0,6	- 0,1	+ 0,45	- 6,681	- 14,847

[1]Cyclophosphamide, Methotrexate and Fluorouracil (anticancer chemotherapy)
[2]Zidovudine (antiretroviral).

Overall survival indicates time to death from any cause. Q-TWIST is an indicator of quality of life. Variations (Δ) on quality of life between two groups (group treated and reference one) are calculated as follows: ΔQ-TWIST = ΔTWIST + U_{AE} x ΔAE + U_{PROG} x ΔPROG where ΔTWIST is a variation on time without symtoms and toxicity. ΔAE is the variation on time spent with adverse events or toxicity. ΔPROG is the variation on time spent in a progressive disease. U_{AE} and U_{PROG} are utility coefficients. They reflect the value of the states of health on a utility scale with reference points 0 and 1:TWIST is assigned a weight of 1 and death a weight of 0. U_{AE} and U_{PROG} were arbitrarily chosen (U_{AE} = U_{PROG} = 0.5) because no patient-derived information was available to indicate the "worth" of life with toxic effects of the treatment or with progression. Six or seven cures of CMF are more suitable for premenopausal women with operable breast cancer than for postmenopausal women (lower cost/Q-TWIST ratios). In the same way, treatment with AZT at 500 mg/day has a better cost-utility ratio than with AZT at 1500 mg/day in HIV patients. This joins the medical decision making that the drug toxicity can be marked (myelosuppression, anaemia, neutropenia, nausea) (10).

With the same hypothesis ($U_{AE} = U_{PROG} = 0,5$), AZT 1 200 mg/day versus placebo during 18 months decreases Q-TWIST to -0,15 months in mildly symptomatic HIV patients (11). In the same way, for AZT 500 mg/day or 1.500 mg/day versus placebo, Q-TWIST falls down to -0,03 and -0,35 months in asymptomatic HIV patients (12). The economic analysis based on cost-utility ratio can not consider these two treatments as efficient. In fact, it joins the clinical decision making which forsaked high dose AZT therapy in mildly symptomatic HIV patients to use AZT at 500 mg/day when clinical conditions are unstable or CD4 count is below 200/mm3 and which delay AZT treatment at least until asymptomatic patients develop symptoms (10).

Most of cancer and AIDS treatments have not yet shown a significant increase in overall survival for patients. They still remain symptomatic or palliative treatments. For this reason and because quality of life is not integrated in the cost/year of life gained unit, the economic analysis based on this value is not adequate for decision making either in cancer or in AIDS.

Cost/QALY and cost/Q-TWIST are more pertinent for economic analysis. They integrate a trade-off between quantity and quality of life. The advantage of measuring quality of life with Q-TWIST model is that it distinguishes three components of quality of life which are relevant with cancer and AIDS non curative treatments:

- Time without symptoms and toxicity
- Time with adverse events or toxicity
- Time with disease progression or relapse

Moreover, Q-TWIST can help economic decision making at the level of the society as well as at the level of the individual: patient-physician relationship. The Q-TWIST model may be applied at an individual scale and allows physician to define for each patient the most efficient treatment.

QUALITY OF LIFE AND EFFICIENCY

Conflicting Objectives?

In the context of the economic evaluation of health programs and treatments, quality of life is considered one of the dimensions of the benefits - of the output - that should be maximised within some given resource constraints. When allocating resources among treatments and patients the costs as well as the benefits should be considered if the general wellbeing of society has to be maximised, because in a world of limited health care resources assigning some resources to a given patient and indication necessarily implies denying its use for another indication or patient. This is precisely the meaning of the economic concept of opportunity cost.

In principle it is in the interest of society that priority is given to those treatments with the best cost-effectiveness ratio, i.e., with a lower cost per QALY, because such a decision rule provides the largest improvement in health from a given amount of resources. This statement is obvious when one consideres distributing these resources to a single patient. However, when one considers the whole population distributional and ethical issues may arise. It is not obvious that society would find it acceptable to deny treatments to a group of patients on the grounds that resources may be more efficiently used - i.e., because more QALYs would be gained - for improving the health of another group of patients. It may well be the case that society attaches a higher priority to treating patients in the worst health conditions even if this implies a smaller global gain in health. This argument is likely to apply to patients with cancer and AIDS.

Economic analysis can provide information on the costs and benefits of treatments that may help decision makers in addressing these difficult issues. But the final decisions require making value judgements which the economic analyst is not legitimately entitled to establish; they are rather the type of political responsibilities that society delegates to its political representatives and decision makers.

REFERENCES

1. Smith RD, Hall J. A cost-utility approach to the use of 5-fluorouracil and levamisole as adjuvant chemotherapy for Dukes' C colonic carcinoma, Med. J. Aust., 1993; 158 : 319–322
2. Hillner BE, Smith TJ. Efficacy and cost-effectiveness of autologous bone marrow transplantation in metastatic breast cancer, JAMA 1992; 267 (15): 2055–61
3. Smith TJ, Hillner BE. The efficacy and cost-effectiveness of adjuvant therapy of early breast cancer in premenopausal women, J. Clin. Oncol., 1993; 11 (4): 771–6
4. Fornander T, Cedemark B, Mattson A, et al. Adjuvant tamoxifen in ealy breast cancer: occurence of new primary cancers, Lancet 1989; 2: 117–20
5. Magriples U, Naftolin F, Schartz PE, et al. High grade endometrial carcinoma in tamoxifen treated breast cancer patients, J. Clin. Oncol.,1993; 11: 485–90
6. Epstein RJ. Does the breast cancer dollar make sense? European Journal of Cancer 1992; 28: 486–91
7. Gelber RD, Goldhirch A, Cavalli F. Quality of life adjusted evaluation of adjuvant therapies for operable breast cancer, An. Int. Med. 1991; 114: 621–28
8. Swanson CE, Tindall B. Efficacy of zidovudine treatment in homosexual men with ARC: factors influencing development of AIDS, survival and drug tolerance, *AIDS*, 1994; 8: 625–34
9. Aboulker JP, Swart AM. Preliminary analysis of the Concorde trial. Correspondence, Lancet 1993; 341: 889–90
10. Barry MG, Back DJ, Breckenridge AM. Zidovudine therapy in HIV infection: which patients should be treated and when, Br. J. Pharmacol., 1995; 40: 107–10
11. Gelber RD, Lederking WR,Cotton DJ, et al. Quality of life evaluation in a clinical trial of zidovudine therapy in patients with midly symptomatic HIV infection, Ann. Int. Med.1992; 116 (12): 961–66
12. Lederking WR, Gelber RD, Cotton DJ, et al. Evaluation of the quality of life associated with zidovudine treatment in asymptomatic human immunodeficiency virus infection, N. Engl. J. Med. *1994; 330: 738–43*
13. Freedberg KA,Tosteson A, Cotton DJ, et al. Optimal management strategies for HIV infected patients who present with cough or dyspnea, J. Gen. Intern. Med., 1992:;7: 261–72
14. Shuman K, Lynn L, Glick H. Cost-effectiveness of ñow dose zidovudine therapy for asymptommatic patients with human immunodeficiency virus (HIV) infection, Ann. Int. Med. 1991; 114/9):798–802

FUTURE ISSUES IN THE USE OF HEALTH STATUS ASSESSMENT MEASURES IN CLINICAL SETTINGS

Sheldon Greenfield, Sherrie H. Kaplan, and Ira B. Wilson

From The Primary Care Outcomes Research Institute
New England Medical Center
750 Washington Street, Box 345
Boston, Massachusetts

Compared to 10 years ago, there is considerable agreement that quality of life is an important aim in the provision of medical care and in the promotion of health. Research in recent years has rendered concrete, meaningful and feasible measures that have turned a vague abstract notion into useful ratings that can find their place alongside mortality, physiologic measures and symptoms in the spectrum of outcomes.

However, as the outcomes movement has quickened pace, the wider and wider application of these measures of Health Related Quality of Life (HRQOL) has met with disappointment. The HRQOL measures, as originally developed, were summary measures of populations, not meant for groups of patients under treatment with specific agents, or for groups of patients cared for in different systems of care, or under different payment mechanisms, or by different providers. Although reliability and feasibility remain high for these measures across widespread applications, the validity becomes more questionable. Since measurement, and therefore the validity of measurement, cannot be devoid of purpose, the central question of this paper is how valid these measures are in their various applications to medical clinical topics such as the success of a drug in AIDS or the success of surgery in cancer. The corollary aim of this paper is to examine ways to retain the central principles of HRQOL measures, but to make them valid and fulfill their purpose in the increasing variety of medical situations in which the generic measures of HRQOL fail to reflect the care provided.

I will focus on three of the major threats to the validity and meaningfulness of these measures. In these three areas major research findings in the last few years have made the use of HRQOL possible in the increasing number of situations in which the concept would otherwise have to be discarded.

The first of these threats is that of case mix, sometimes referred to as severity of illness, but in reality encompassing all the confounders that would bias a relationship between the treatment (defined broadly as a drug, an educational program, a geographic

Cancer, AIDS, and Quality of Life, edited by Levy *et al.*
Plenum Press, New York, 1997

area, a type of provider, a type of health system, a type of payment, any independent variable) and the outcome, HRQOL. This factor addresses the non specificity of the HRQOL measures. Research has demonstrated that the general measures of HRQOL are profoundly affected by the variety of factors: socioeconomic status, age, prior functional status, and severity of illness, which importantly includes not just the disease or tracer being studied, but also the severity of the coexistent conditions.

Numerous recent studies illustrate the non trivial effect of illness severity on the interpretation of outcome results. It is important to anchor discussions of illness severity adjustment with examples of comparisons of mortality rates, which, it is now appreciated, would be unthinkable without adjustment. In fact, risk adjusted mortality is referred to as a "model" where, in a multivariate manner, all of the potential confounders are included simultaneously in the prediction of death. The case of Coronary Artery Bypass Graft (CABG) mortality is the best developed, and with work of Hannan[1] and O'Conner,[2] are among the best examples. Also, there have several recent examples of risk adjusted mortality for chronic disease, using measures of comorbid diseases as the adjustor. One of the best is that of prostate cancer in work by Albertson et al,[3] where 10 year mortality was as much affected by the patient's comorbid conditions, summarized by an index called "ICED", as by the tumor stage. Similarly, in an observational study of mortality following either transurethral prostatectomy and open prostatectomy, various comorbidity measures were compared with respect to their ability to predict mortality. Mortality differences between the procedures, found in earlier studies, were not present after adjustment for comorbidity at baseline, using these indexes.[4]

HRQOL measures arose out of a social science framework, but considering the fact that so many medical conditions, symptoms, and laboratory abnormalities affect functional status, it is, perhaps, surprising that unique "risk adjusted functional status" models are not developed for each medical condition. In patients with diabetes, for example, the average score on the Short Form-36 Physical Function Index is 67, but, scores vary by large amounts (85 to 47) according to medical illness severity using a newly developed patient based method of reporting of symptoms and disease manifestations.[5] If two drugs, cities, systems or whatever were being compared, and they had different distributions of baseline illness severity, they would experience different HRQOL outcomes that would be due to illness rather than the intervention.

Kaplan et al found that same phenomenon in patients recovering from either laparoscopic or traditional cholecystectomy.[6] The HRQOL outcomes at 3 months were affected in a major way by medical illness severity. Similarly, AIDS and cancer patients may have a distinct set of medical comorbidities. Without control for these, results could be biased.

A recent study showed that the index described above, developed by aggregating symptoms and disease manifestations into a scaled index, better predicted HRQOL outcomes than a list of diagnoses. In two patient samples, one poor and one middle class, the diagnosis list was comparable (4.4 to 3.0), but the distribution of severity was very different when using an index which is more sensitive than the list.[7] This new index explained 33% of the variance in future functional status, vs 24% with a list. A recent international comparison of HRQOL outcomes of patient with AMI, was flawed because, a small difference in the functional status score could have been due to twice as much comorbidity in the Canadian sample compared to the American sample.[8] A full review of the issues and principles of case mix can be found in a recent publication.[9]

A second issue is sensitivity. Many investigators have complained that certain side effects of treatments may be important to patients, but not reflect themselves in general HRQOL measures (e.g., ability to walk, keep a job, take care of children etc.). A study by

Litwin et al of prostate cancer showed that illness stage and treatment affected what they called "bother" but not the general measures. In a study of BPH, surgery did not change the level of general health status, but it markedly affected the patient's symptoms.[10] In a recent unpublished study by Kaplan et al, diabetes specific measures, termed "hassles", were more related to treatment regimen than physical function. An earlier study, using items from rheumatoid arthritis, showed similar results: specific hassles correlated better with joint count than did the general measures. The work by Kaplan attempts to make the disease specific measure generalizable, by creating dimensions such as hassles, body image, worry etc. that are common to all conditions, while having items that are specific to a disease. These measures also correlate at low levels with generic measures. Without disease specific measures, important intervention differences will be missed.

The final issue surrounds the link between process and outcome. In discussing this, there arise two perspectives, which are often polarized. One is that outcomes can stand by themselves: the presentation of information on poor outcomes should galvanize action aimed at finding out what went wrong. Correction of what went wrong would lead to improved outcomes. Implicit in this view is that medical processes and the multivariate elements that go into care, from nursing encouragement to timely arrival of medications to physician decision making, are too complex to allow identification of the one thing that went wrong, the one guideline not followed. The other view is that outcomes without systematic process measurement are not useful; if the outcomes are poor, they can only be improved by letting the physician or provider know exactly which processes were at fault. This latter emphasis leads to process or guidelines development, with outcomes serving as the research base for constructing the guidelines. It is easy to see why polarization could occur, but it is also easy to envision the synthesis of the two positions, with both or alternating processes and outcomes leading the evaluations.

Three studies exemplify this sought after bond between processes and HRQOL. One is a study of asthma by Haas et al in which better technical outcomes and more appropriate drug therapy led to better functional status.[11] Another effort, by Kaplan and Greenfield et al, in several studies, found a link between interpersonal care of the physician and functional status.[12] More specifically, when the patients were more active in the doctor patient conversation and when the physician encouraged increased participation, the functional status of the patient was better. Finally, the recently reported study of Wilson et al, found that the presence and severity of certain symptom complexes in patients with AIDS were directly related, in multivariate analyses, to functional outcomes.[13] The implication of this kind of finding is that while physicians should do whatever they can for these patients, that they should be sure to include a focus on alleviating certain symptoms, for which they and their patient will be rewarded with improved patient reported HRQOL. These three studies, resting on three different aspects of processes (drug therapy, interpersonal care, and the focus on specific symptoms in specific diseases) all point to the need to go as far as possible in determining linkages between processes and outcomes. The measurement of HRQOL need not await research into the links and can stand by itself to evaluate and improve care, but the identification of those links increase the chances of improving care.

As these three areas, case mix, disease-specific HRQOL and process-outcome links are investigated and clarified, other issues that need to be dealt with, will arise: the correct time interval between the provision of care and the assessment of HRQOL; the role of patient characteristics beyond the health provider's control; the role of provider characteristics, such as provider satisfaction; the meaning of HRQOL in special populations such as children; the costs of obtaining HRQOL measurement on a routine basis; all of these will loom as challenges for future research.[14,15] Meanwhile, we are closer to the goal of using HRQOL to evaluate and optimize care, to balance costs against that optimization, and to enhance the patient's role as a partner in the delivery of health services.

REFERENCES

1. Hannan EL, Kilburn H, Racz M, et al. Improving the outcomes of coronary artery bypass surgery in New York State. *JAMA*. 271(10):761–766, 1994.
2. O'Connor GT, et al. A regional prospective study of in-hospital mortality associated with coronary artery bypass grafting. *JAMA*. 1991;266(6):803–809.
3. Albertson PC, Fryback DG, Storer BE, Kolon TF, Fine H. Long-term survival among men with conservatively treated localized prostate cancer. *JAMA*. 1995;274(8):626–631.
4. Krousel-Wood MA, Abdoh A, Re R. Comparing comorbid-illness indices assessing outcome variation: The case of prostatectomy. *Journal of General Internal Medicine*. 1996;11:32–38.
5. Greenfield S, Sullivan L, Dukes KA, Silliman R, D'Agostino R, Kaplan SH. Development and Testing of a New Measure of Case-Mix for Use in Office Practice. *Medical Care*. Vol 33(4):AS47-AS57, April, 1995.
6. Kaplan SH, Shea J, Khan A, Dukes KA, Bachwich D, Escarce J, Clark J, Schwartz JS, Greenfield S. The impact of surgery vs. non-operative treatment on the health outcomes of gallstone patients: Results from the Biliary Tract Disease Patient Outcomes Research Team. *In preparation*.
7. Greenfield S, Dukes KA, Sullivan L, Kaplan SH. Under estimation of severity of illness in the urban poor. *In preparation*.
8. Mark DB, Naylor CD, Hlatky MA, et al. Use of medical resources and quality of life after acute myocardial infarction in Canada and the United States. *NEJM*. 331:1130–1135, 1994.
9. Greenfield S, Sullivan LM, Silliman RA, et al. Principles and practice of case mix adjustment: Applications to end-stage renal disease. *Am J Kid Dis*. 24(2):298–307, 1994.
10. Epstein RS, Deverka PA, Chute CG, et al. Validation of a new quality of life questionnaire for benign prostatic hyperplasia. *Journal of Clinical Epidemiology*. 45(12):1431–1445, 1992.
11. Haas JS, Cleary PD, Guadagnoli E, et al. The Impact of Socioeconomic Status on the Intensity of ambulatory Treatment and Health Outcomes after Hospital Discharge for Adults with Asthma. *Journal of General Internal Medicine*. March 1994;(9):121–126.
12. Kaplan SH, Greenfield S, Ware JE, Jr., Assessing the effects of physician-patient interactions on the outcomes of chronic disease. *Medical Care*. 27(3):S110-S127, 1989.
13. Wilson IB, Cleary PD. Clinical predictors of functioning in persons with acquired immune deficiency syndrome. *Medical Care*, In Press.
14. Deyo RA, Patrick DL. Barriers to the use of health status measures in clinical investigation, patient care, and policy research. *Medical Care*, 1989;27(3):S254- S268.
15. Greenfield S, Nelson E. Recent development and future issues in the use of health status assessment measures in clinical settings. *Medical Care*, 1992;30(5S):23–41.

10

QUALITY OF LIFE AT THE END STAGES OF LIFE

Daniel Callahan

Rhone-Poulenc Rorer Inc.
500 Arcola Rd.
PO Box 1200
Collegeville, Pennsylvania 19246

Death has never been easy for human beings. The meaning of death is now and has always been a profound mystery. As if that has not been difficult enough, the transition from death to life has unsettled all but the most hardy spirits. The enormous and troubling irony of modern death, however, is that medicine seems to have made it harder, not easier, to die. Perhaps that is not surprising. The premise of modern scientific medicine is that, with sufficient knowledge and skill, death and illness can be overcome, pushed aside at least for a time, and perhaps for a longer and longer time.

There is much evidence to support that premise: lives can be extended now in a way that would have been inconceivable even a few decades ago. I recently saw a film that featured three American women in their mid-seventies talking about their wonderfully successful liver transplants; and not long after that I visited a hospital that boasted of its success in putting a pacemaker in a 104-year-old patient. Many people with AIDS, who would have died quickly a decade ago, are still alive today because of an array of advances that have learned better how to cope with the disease. Many children who in earlier times would have died of cancer are now being saved; and the 85-year-old mother of my wife recently had a most successful operation to remove cancerous breast tumors.

The great problem in all of this is that life at the borderline of life and death has become more, not less difficult. How can this be? Don't we know more than ever about the relief of pain and suffering? Don't we have greater and greater skills in prognosis? Don't we have more and more public and professional discussion about the end of life, and how to improve the quality of that end? Has not death, and the care of the dying, seen an explosive burst of books, conferences, educational programs, and new forms of care (such as the hospice movement)? Despite all of these developments, there is not only considerable medical uneasiness about the care of the dying, but considerable public discomfort as well.

I want to try to understand this phenomenon by looking at three aspects of the quality of life at the end of life. One of them bears on the doctor-patient relationship and the

Cancer, AIDS, and Quality of Life, edited by Levy *et al.*
Plenum Press, New York, 1997

right of patients to know the truth about their illness and their prognosis. The second bears
on the training of physicians, nurses, and other health care workers to enhance the quality
of life of their dying patients. The third aspect, particularly intriguing, is the way modern
medicine understands its relationship to death, which brings us, I believe, to the heart of
our problem.

1. DOCTORS, PATIENTS, AND TRUTH-TELLING

The husband of a French friend of mine recently died of cancer in a Parisian hospital. "How was it?" I asked her rather hesitantly. She was angry and a little bitter. It was
not just the cancer that made his last days difficult, but the silence, and human unrespon-
siveness, of the doctors. "We were told nothing," she said, and could not get their questions answered. I thought such stories were unique to the United States, but they are
common throughout the world. Modern patients want to hear the truth—not all of them of
course, but a growing number—and they have a right to the truth.

The ancient traditions of medical ethics, going back to Hippocrates, had as one of
their goals that of preserving hope in patients. This came to be interpreted by physicians
as the necessity to lie to patients, or to evade the truth, if that seemed the only way to
maintain hope. This was always thought particularly necessary in the case of cancer, a
particularly dread disease. That was not necessarily a bad philosophy when physicians
could do comparatively little to preserve life. But it makes little sense these days, when
physicians can do more, when patients are better educated, and when there are difficult
choices that must be made.

We should, moreover, have a better appreciation now about the other side of the
coin labeled lying and deception to spare patients anxiety; that is, that uncertainty and a
lack of knowledge and a distrust of physician veracity can also engender anxiety. The evidence is increasingly strong from many countries that those patients who want to be told
the truth do not in fact collapse or despair at being given bad news. They are often in a
better position to cope with their condition—and have a good relationship with their doctor than when lying was the standard practice. Naturally, there will be some people who
will either say directly, or give unmistakable signs, that they would rather not hear bad
news. That should be respected as well. A good quality of life with terminal illness will be
one that is marked by a relationship of sensitivity and equality between doctor and patients. Truth-telling, for those who want it, is a symbol of equality.

2. THE CARE OF THE DYING

Training and Sensitivity

If there is any universal truth about the training of physicians, it is that practically
nowhere is systematic attention given to the care of the dying and the quality of life of the
terminally ill. Even in a number of those countries that now include such issues in courses
on medical ethics as a part of medical education, it is rarely followed up or implemented
during the clinical training of young physicians. It is said that, as far back as the time of
the Greeks, doctors fled when death was at hand, sometimes to avoid the imputation of
failure, but more often because they felt there was nothing more for them to do.

Efforts have been made in recent decades to change such attitudes and the practice of silence about death during clinical training. It has not been easy. The potent scientific bias of medical education, the failure even to teach basic communication skills, the uneasiness that doctors along with everyone else feel in the presence of death and dying, all contribute to the widespread failure of doctors to deal well with death. When to that basic problem is added the general ethos of modern hospitals, oriented to aggressive, high-technology treatment, it is hardly any wonder that dying is handled so poorly. No one quite knows what to do with it, and the most common response is to flee, as common now as 2500 years ago.

The hospice movement, which began in Great Britain in the late 1960s and which has spread gradually to a number of other countries as well, was meant to bring about a fundamental change in that situation. Its goal has been to train people specifically to care for the dying, beginning with a capacity simply to talk with them, and then honing their skills in palliative medicine and the relief of pain and suffering, and doing those things either at home or in special institutions devoted to the care of the dying. These programs—heavily oriented to cancer patients but now extending out to include those with AIDS and other terminal conditions as well—have been enormously successful.

Yet how strange it is, when one thinks of it, that modern medicine has had to invent a special institution and set of practices to care for the dying—and to do so out of the mainstream of technological medicine. Should not this be a part of ordinary and routine medicine? It should, but that is not the case and, however odd, it is a good thing that at least some people in medicine have tried to find satisfactory alternatives to the kinds of high-technology death that so often lack any sensitivity to the quality of life of patients at the end of life.

I first became aware of this lack some years ago while accompanying a group of physicians on rounds in an intensive care unit. It was quite clear that the machines and instruments and gauges held far more interest for the doctors than the patients to whom they were attached. For evey minute where there was eye-to-eye contact between doctor and patient, much less conversation, there were five where the only eye-to-eye contact was with the machines. I can hardly help recalling as well the death of my own mother. Just a few days before her death, while she was still quite alert and talkative, her physician managed to talk with me for 15 minutes in her hospital room without once talking to her or even looking at her. I might add that she was suffering from cancer of the colon, a disease that had killed her mother and a sister and which she had feared all of her life. She did not ask if she had cancer, and there seemed no reason in that case to tell her. But even a physician who decides that, in some cases, it is wiser to withhold the truth should never withhold his eyes from his patient.

3. MEDICINE AND DEATH

The Great Schism

At the heart of modern medicine there is, I believe, a fundamental schism about death, suggesting that medicine simply has not been able to find a proper stance toward it. I would describe this schism as the struggle between two very different responses to the problem of death, and with it the response to terminally ill patients.

There is, on the hand, and particularly in compassionate clinical medicine, the understanding that death is a part of life, that all every person and every patient eventually dies. That is a our biological fate, shared with all other organic beings. Sensitive clinical medicine works to enhance the possibility of a peaceful death, one in particular not marked by an excessive and destructive effort to prolong life no matter what the cost. Death comes to us all and medicine must make its peace with death.

There is, on the other hand however, research medicine. For that medicine death remains the great enemy, and modern medical research has targeted each and every cause of death for eradication. It is not, I suppose, that researchers really believe that immortality can be had through medical progress, but they do seem to believe that all of the causes of death are, in effect, biological accidents, contingent events that can be overcome with greater scientific understanding and technological innovation. For the zealous researcher—eager to find a cure for cancer, or AIDS, or heart disease, or the dementias—death is not an acceptable part of life at all; it is outside of, and hostile to, life. If immortality is not anyone's intention, that is the implicit logic of the research enterprise. For medical research, there is no peace to be made with death: it is the enemy, to be attacked with all possible zeal.

The schism I refer to now comes clearly into view: medicine is a house divided in its understanding of the place of death in life. Part of medicine tries to live with and accommodate death, while another part will have nothing to do with that stance. Even the clinical level becomes infected with the research attitude. Doctors often feel they have failed when patients die, even when they rationally know that there is nothing they could have done. The aggressive stance toward death assumes that, with good enough medicine, and better research, death might be averted. By making death a repairable biological accident, the research stance overflows into the clinical arena. Doctors themselves often see the death of a patient as either a failure of theirs or a failure of medicine, or perhaps both.

This schism at the heart of medicine also affects patients and the general public. There are almost everywhere unrealistic expectations about medicine: patients expect miracles, and they are often bitter when medicine can not produce them. Partly because it is of the nature of research to be optimistic, and partly because the media and the public is drawn to the drama of medical progress, hope is always high and expectations enormous.

The quality of life at the end of life is often the victim of the schism. Neither patients nor physicians are quite sure whether death is friend or enemy, to be accepted or fought, and whether the medical thrust should be toward aggressive treatment or palliative care only. Cancer provides the most telling example of this struggle. Cancer research and therapy has long been one of the most aggressive theaters of medical aspiration. It is marked by high hopes, large amounts of money, and tremendous patient pressures. There is a powerful inclination not to give in to the disease, to pursue even the most marginal possibilities of a cure or remission, and to bury realistic appraisals under layers of optimism, real or feigned. In the case of cancer also, clinician and researcher are often one and the same, particular in the major teaching and research centers.

Given that general ambience, it is hardly surprising that good palliative care for cancer patients has always taken second place to the drive for treatment. We know from survey after survey over the past two or three decades that too few physicians are well trained in palliative medicine, in oncology as well as other specialties. If you examine the major American medical textbook, *Cecil Textbook on Medicine*, you will see that the lengthy section on cancer has not a word about palliative care when the fight against the disease has been lost. For that matter, the entire section says hardly a word about the fact that large numbers of cancer patients die. I suspect the textbooks in other countries display the same tendencies.

The World Health Organization's unit on cancer and palliative care, moreover, has amply documented the extent to which expensive, acute care medicine for cancer patients often leaves no room, or money, for palliative care. This has become especially true in many developing countries, where entire cancer budgets are devoted to high-technology treatments—usually started too late because the patients arrive too late—and even the most basic palliative care drugs are not even available, either because they are illegal or because no money is budgeted for them. Death is the great enemy, but it seems utterly forgotten that death will come to vast numbers of cancer patient. When death from cancer is made the only or major enemy, then the stage is set to threaten the quality of life of those who will die from cancer.

THE STRUGGLE FOR A PEACEFUL DEATH

There are two fundamental elements that will influence the quality of life at the end of life. One is external, the other internal. The external element is the way in which the critically ill or dying patient is treated by others. Is there empathy, sensitivity, competent palliative care, and an appropriate shifting of attention and emphasis away from cure and toward the enhancement of a good death? It is the unwillingness to accept death, to give up the search for a cure, that is often the enemy of a peaceful death. There can be, in this world, an excess of misplaced virtue, and the desire to save life when the odds are heavily against that, can be such a case.

Medicine's drive to cure, to save, to rehabilitate is a virtue, but it is not a virtue to be blind to those circumstances which indicate that the quest is hopeless, that a different course and direction are needed. We should be enormously ambivalent about modern medicine's great strength: its drive to conquer nature, to bring it to heel, to overpower it. In death medicine always meets its match, and the great need is to see when death can no longer be held at bay, when it will finally exert its ultimate dominion. If it is the saving of life alone that is thought to be the only or supreme value, then we can be sure that the quality of life will suffer. A death excessively resisted is a death likely to be far harder, far more of an assault on a patient's dignity, than one which is accepted and worked with.

Yet it is important here to recognize that the quality of a patient's dying will have much to do with the patient himself. This is the internal element of dying. As the great essayist Michel de Montaigne once wrote: "Fortune appears somewhat purposely to wait for the last years of our lives in order to show us she can overthrow in one moment what she has taken long years to build....In this last scene between ourselves and death, there is no more pretence. We must use plain words, and display such goodness or purity as we have at the bottom of the pot." The great seventeenth-century English theologian Jeremy Taylor made a similar point: "be ready for it [death] by the preparation of a good life....Else there is nothing that can comfort you....For if you fear death, you shall never the more avoid it, but you make it miserable....No man can be a slave but that he fears pain, or fears to die."

All of this is only to say that, if we are to have a death with dignity, a death that reflects a sensitivity to the quality of life, we will have to supply much of that ourselves. The most that others can do, from the outside and externally, is to be with us, to make the physical, and psychological, and spiritual conditions as beneficent as possible. After that, we will be on our own. At this point, many of us will be ambivalent, uncertain what is required of us: acceptance of death, or a struggle to the end against death? This ambivalence is seen with great frequency in the care of cancer and AIDS patients: to fight or to give in? To accept death or to deny death?

In my country—and I would expect most other places as well—we commend the cancer or AIDS patient who is a fighter, who searches with singleminded dedication for a cure or remission. But we also, ironically, no less commend the patient who graciously accepts death, who does not put up a fight. Well, which ideal do we want to cultivate? No wonder that so many patients are uncertain how to respond to their disease: that medicine which treats them is itself ambivalent and torn, and that ambivalence has been well communicated to the general public.

I can offer no simple way to resolve this ambivalence other than to say this: we are not likely to die well, much less peacefully, if we have not prior to our dying come to accept death as our fate and part of our human condition. And we are likely to make our death all the more difficult if we insist upon perfect control. The drive for control of nature and disease has been at the heart of modern scientific medicine; and that has been a source of its power and its success. But when the desire for control runs wild, when that desire itself gets (so to speak) out of control, then harmful consequences are likely to follow. For our dying is the ultimate loss of control, when our body turns fully against us and would return us to the dust from which we came. It is hard to see how there can be a good quality of life at the end of life if we insist on maintaining perfect control of that end.

There is now a strong movement in some countries, including my own, to make legal euthanasia or physician-assisted suicide, or both. I can not take up that controversy here, nor lay out my reasons for opposing that movement. I will only observe that its main characteristic is an obsession with control. That is surely understandable in one way: the fear of a loss of control is a basic part of the fear of death. But the movement also looks suspiciously like an effort to make good on the failure of medicine itself successfully to control with science and technology our life and death. Its control has turned out to be partial only, and there seems little or no likelihood that it will ever utterly subdue or human nature and human biology. Euthanasia or physician-assisted suicide seems meant to fill in the gap, to get one wayh or another the perfection of control that medicine with all of its sophisticated skills has not quite been able to bring us. It is a movement that promises to put fate back into our own hands.

I believe that is a false promise, simply magnifying the original mistake of an overly ambitious medicine in thinking it could master our fate. It no less fails to understand that the quality of life at the end of life is not just a matter of mastering the external circumstances of death, in this case that of bringing death at just the moment we want it and on our own terms. Montaigne and Taylor were right in thinking that it is the kind of life we live, and what we bring to our death from that life, which will be the main determinant of the quality of our death.

There has been much talk of late about "rational suicide." I suppose that is possible as a theoretical idea. The evidence nonetheless indicates that the overwhelming majority of those who commit suicide—and thus are in the future likely to want the help of their physician to do so—have had a previous history of depression. They bring to their death, so often sad and an expression of despair, not the problem of finding a meaning in death but of finding a meaning for a life that has been long lost.

What, in the end, is a peaceful death, a death that can be said to enhance as much as possible the quality of life of the dying patient? I would define such a death as one where, first of all, the dying person herself is reconciled to death—not to its goodness surely, but at least to its inevitability. It is also, ideally, a death that has been preceded by reflection on one's life, and an effort to prepare that life for death, getting things right, to use Montaigne's phrase, "at the bottom of the pot." It should no less be a death in the company of the living, who will gather about us—whether our medical caretakers or our family and friends—to accompany us to death and to lend whatever support they can. To speak ideally once again, death should be preceded by consciousness as close to the time of death as possible (and only relinquished for the relief of unbearable pain), to allow interaction with others and with oneself.

A peaceful death will be one that doctors seek for their patients. This will only be possible—or at least enhanced as a possibility—if doctors recognize that the care of their patients in their dying is just as important as they care they can give to keep them alive. Every physician who must treat a dying patient ought to be one for whom there is a strong and lively tension between a desire to keep the patient away from death and a desire not to deform the dying of the patient. The overwhelming tendency now in medicine is to worry more about keeping patients alive than in worrying about how they will die. The latter is too often seen as something added on, a second-best choice when treatment has failed.

That is the wrong stance. All patients will eventually die, and the most successful treatments only defer death to a later time or a different disease. Death always wins in the long run, and the physician who keeps this in mind, who knows that how he accompanies his patient to death will matter as much to the quality of life of that patient as anything previously done, will at least be on the right track. I am not suggesting here that patients too easily be allowed to die. What I am looking for is a dynamic tension, where the struggle for life is balanced by a struggle for a good death.

In the end, medicine can not guarantee any patient a good death, nor can we guarantee one to ourselves by the way we think about and approach our death. What we can do much better, however, is to put death back into medicine, to stop treating it as the ultimate enemy. It may well be *an* ultimate enemy. But to make it *the* ultimate enemy is to fail to respect our human nature. We die. That is the way things are. Medicine needs to better understand that fact, the same medicine which has worked to rid us of all the causes of death and which can not find a place for the dying in its textbooks.

Cancer and AIDS are indeed enemies of life. But they are also the way many of us are going to die. If in our zeal to destroy them as enemies, we forget that they are also causes of death—and all death must have a cause—then they will truly have bettered us. That need not be the case.

11

QUALITY OF LIFE

The Experience of an Oncology Unit Functioning in a Rural Greek Area

Vassilis Georgoulias, Charalaubos Kourousis, and Stelios Kakolyris

Department of Medical Oncology
School of Medicine, University of Crete
University General Hospital of Crete, PO Box 1352
711 10 Heraklion, Crete, Greece

INTRODUCTION

Each individual has the essential right to health. This right is recognized, in a general manner, by the Universal Declaration of Human Rights, but also by the International Conventions concerning civil, political, social and cultural rights. In the latter case, in particular, article 12 provides that the States, which are party to the convention, recognize the right for each individual to enjoy the best physical and mental state of health, which one is capable to achieve.

To reach the above goals, measures must be taken by the States but also by the responsible physicians and the patients' familial enviroment. However, the tremendous evolution of the biomedical science and medical technology, during the last decades, created several bioethical problems. Indeed, one of the most mportant moral and social values is that the patient is not a simple biological unit, but a personality and a vehicle of dignity. The responsible physicians have not to forget that the target of their actions is not only the disease but also the patient who must be protected and cured with dignity and respect. These important parameters should be ensured by both the physicians and the patients' familial enviroment.

The majority of patients with widespead common cancers will not be cured by local or other treatments. For these patients, the purpose of medical care is to prolong their lives. Nevertheless, both the disease progession and the applied treatments - conventional or experimental - may have deleterious effects on the quality of life. Thus, the overall benefit from a treatment is often uncertain. However, in several cases a specific treatment could be partially successful producing remarkable and, sometimes, durable relief of symptoms.

Cancer, AIDS, and Quality of Life, edited by Levy *et al.*
Plenum Press, New York, 1997

Table 1. Problems to be confronted after a diagnosis of cancer has been
established in the Cretan population

Problems	Frequency (%)
Usefulness of any therapeutic intervention	50
Effectiveness of the treatment	30
Objections to the diagnosis	90
Treatment–related toxicity	40
Patients' psycho-social problems	40

The management of cancer patients by an antineoplastic treatment requires the estableshment of trust between the patient and physician. This could be achieved by a honest communication between the two involved parties, i. e. the patient and the responsible physician. There is no clear method to establish a reliable confidence with the cancer patient especially in cases where a definitive cure doesn't exist. Therefore, the diagnosis of cancer is a real reason of frightening both patients and their family enviroment. The acceptance of the diagnosis of cancer by each individual patient depends on several factors such as their philosophical significance of the truth, the patients' capability to accept the new status of their health, and the physicians' capacity to evaluate the patients' psychological reserves. These problems are further complicated by the fact that doctors have to explain to their patients not only the perspectives of their disease or the side effects of the different therapeutic procedures but, also, the painful and difficult medical situations which could be presented during the evolution of their disease.

It is obvious that this establishment of confidence and trust between the patient and physician is based on the objective and truthful patients' information. There is no doubt that this is one of the most difficult tasks of the physician as well as one of the most important rights of the patient and nobody can deprive them from it. It is also well known that the honest information on the patient can facilitate their compliance to treatment and, in general, the management of their disease.

Several reports have shown that the number of physicians who announce the diagnosis of cancer is increasing and, in several countries, this practice is routine. However, several patients cannot accept the truth. This is mainly due, as stated above, to the patients' prersonality but also to their philosophical and cultural background. Moreover, an important factor is the patients' familial environment which, frequently, acts as a shield between the patient and the doctor.

This problem is still important in Greece and, especially, to regions outside the important urban areas. Greeks, as a Mediterannean people, are characterized by sentimental reactions when faced by severe health problems. The patients' relatives frequently believe that good service is offered to the patients if no announcement of the diagnosis is made.

RESULTS AND DISCUSSION

We evaluated the question of patients' information about the diagnosis of cancer in the Department of Medical Oncology of the University of Crete. This Department covers the whole island of the rural area of Crete with 600.000 inhabitants. About 70% of the population occupies the agricultural sector and, therefore, their educational level is relatively low. Indeed, 18% of the island population is University or post - College certified. The educational levvel is equivalent to High School / College and Elementary School in 50% and 30%, respectively. Conversely, only 2% are illiterate.

This relatively low educational level as well as the low level of health education of the people from Crete has important impacts on the problems encountered in 2500 cancer patients observed in our Department since 1991. Indeed, in 90% of the cases the patients' relatives were opposed or have serious objections to the announcement of the diagnosis to the patient. The second notable point is that both patients and their relatives believe that once the diagnosis of a neoplastic disease has been made, any therapeutic effort is in vain since no radical treatment for the disease is available. Finally, only one third of the patients are preoccupied by the treatment effectiveness or toxicity in addition to their psycho - social problems.

At diagnosis, 35% of our patients were clearly informed. In almost all the cases, the patients demanded the truth and the discussion with their responsible physician. In addition, 30% of the patients were partially informed by their physicians. In this particular case, the patient is informed that suffers from a precancereous condition with an abnormal cell proliferation which needs a specific treatment in order to prevent its evolution to a fullblown cancer. This intermediate situation was chosen in order to overcome the objections of patients' relatives and, in our experience, it prepares the patient to accept the diagnosis during the treatment procedure. Although we have not investigated whether such explanations are really believed by the patients, the estimation of the treating physicians is that patients feel more comfortable and accept this information without believing it. Finally, 40% of the patients dont know the diagnosis, although half of them have serious suspicions, obtained by the hospital environment or other patients.

An important proportion of the patients, however, obtain the full information about their disease from the medical staff during the treatment period. Indeed, a definitive diagnosis could be announced in 80% of the partially informed patients and in 70% of the patients which have serious suspicions. Conversely, only half of those who ignore their diagnosis obtain information either directly or indirectly. Overall, we can estimate that about 75 - 80% of our patients know the definitive diagnosis at the end of their treatment.

An interesting question was the relationship between the psychological acceptance of the real diagnosis and the patients' educational level. We observed that the procedure of acceptance is directly related to the patients' educational level. Eighty per cent and 62% of the University and High School / College - certified patients accept the diagnosis of cancer, respectively; conversely, the corresponding proportions were 47% and 40% for the Elementary School - certified and illiterate patients, respectively. However, the patients' compliance with the treatment was partially correlated with their educational level. Indeed, Table 2 shows that more than 70% of the patients accepted the treatment, irrespec-

Table 2. Patients' compliance with the treatment according to their educational level

Educational level	Compliance
Illiterate	73%
Elementary school	77%
High school/college	82%
University	90%

Table 3. Reasons to refuse/discontinus treatment according to the patients' information level

Reasons	Fully Informed	Partially Informed	Serious Suspicions	Lack of Information
Diagnosis	11%	14%	21%	33%
Progression of disease	5%	8%	15%	25%
Treatment–related toxicity	15%	22%	3%	5%
Pain	1%	4%	10%	24%
Concommitant diseases	3%	3%	5%	2%

tive of their educational level. However, the compliance was higher in the high educated group of patients, reaching 90% in the University / College - certified patients.

Table 3 presents the reasons leading patients to discontinue treatment according to the status of their initial information. Fully and partially informed patients mainly refuse to continue treatment because of its toxicity (15% and 22%, respectively; Table 3). Conversely, patients ingnoring their diagnosis refuse to continue treatment because of disease progression (25%) or the painfull syndromes which fail to be relieved by the treatment (24%) (Table 3). It is noteworthy that treatment - related toxicity does not represent and important factor for the treatment discontinuation in patients who have a good level of information (15% and 22% for the fully and partially informed, respectively; Table 3). Since the information level is directly related to the educational level, we anticipate that the refusal of treatment might also be related to the patients' educational level.

CONCLUSION

These data strongly suggest that the acceptance of the diagnosis of cancer in a Greek rural area is, mainly, related to the patients' educational level. Moreover, an important number of noninformed patients have the full information about their diagnosis during the treatment procedure by the medical staff. The knoweledge of the diagnosis is strongly related with the patients' compliance with the treatment; however, the educational level also seems to be an important factor for the patients' compliance with the treatment.

A major problem observed in the medical practice and, confirmed in our study, was the lack of information of the Cretan population about the therapeutic possibilities in cancer as well as the probality of achieving long term remission and cure this disease. This is mainly due to the lack of health education, in general, in Greece. Therefore, it is urgent to initiate, by both the governmental and non-governmental instutition, an information campaign of the population in order to communicate the recent advances of medical oncology and biomedical science. Although the diagnosis of cancer is frightening for each patient, the knowledge that some types of cancer could be prevented or, even, cured could increase the patients' confidence to the medicine and facilitate their treatment.

12

ADVOCACY FOR PATIENTS WITH CANCER QUALITY OF LIFE IMPLICATIONS

Joan Marks

Health Advocacy Program
Sarah Lawrence College
Bronxville, New York 10708

The Genetic Revolution is having a profound effect on medical care today. Nowhere is that influence more significant than in the area of cancer care. Our understanding of the genetic basis of cancer and the discovery of "cancer prone genes" has changed our approach to the services and options available to cancer patients and those options can have a major influence on Quality of Life issues. Patients around the world are concerned about how genes may control their cancer destiny.

If a family history is positive and adequate documentation of cancer is made in a family, the patient needs to be informed about his or her personal risk for cancer. Management strategies need to be outlined and preventive options discussed. If DNA testing is available, a thorough explanation of the procedure along with the risks, both psychological and medical, need to be reviewed in detail. Without extensive counseling and a review of options, informed consent cannot be exercised by the patient or family.

The Patient's Bill of Rights issues by the American Hospital (1), provided a set of guidelines to publicly affirm the quality of care patients could expect in health care institutions. In the United States today, hospitals must be accredited by the Joint Commission on Accreditation of Hospitals (JCAHO)(2) and the JCAHO requires that the Patient's Bill of Rights be distributed to patients and the sixteen items on the Bill be guaranteed to all patients. Recently, hospitals in France have also adopted a Bill of Rights.

Implicit in the exercise of the Patient's Bill of Rights is the role of the consumer as his/her own advocate. But the diagnosis of cancer or AIDS places patients in a situation of extreme vulnerability and reduced ability to cope. Patients at these times also need someone to advocate *for* them and to share the burden of all the information gathering that enables patients to make informed decisions about their care.

Since 1969, Sarah Lawrence College in Bronxville, New York (a suburb of New York City) has offered a masters degree to train non-physician genetic counselors. Over 500 genetic counselors, representing nearly half of the trained counselors in the United States have graduated from this program and have been certified by the American Board of Medical Genetics. A rigorous curriculum and extensive on-the-job training have com-

Cancer, AIDS, and Quality of Life, edited by Levy *et al.*
Plenum Press, New York, 1997

Table 1. Patient's Bill of Rights

1. Understand and use these rights. If for any reason you do not understand or you need help, the hospital must provide assistance, including an interpreter.
2. Receive treatment without discrimination as to race, color, religion, sex, national origin, disability, sexual orientation, or source of payment.
3. Receive considerate and respectful care in a clean and safe environment free of unnecessary restraints.
4. Receive emergency care if you need it.
5. Be informed of the name and position of the doctor who will be in charge of your care in the hospital.
6. Know the name, positions, and functions of any hospital staff involved in your care and refuse their treatment, examination or observation.
7. A no smoking room.
8. Receive complete information about your diagnosis, treatment and prognosis.
9. Receive all the information that you need to give informed consent for any proposed procedure or treatment. This information shall include the possible risks and benefits of the procedure or treatment.
10. Receive all the information you need to give informed consent for an order not to resuscitate. You also have the right to designate an individual to give this consent for you if you are too ill to do so. If you would like additional information, please ask for a copy of the pamphlet "Do Not Resuscitate Orders - A Guide for Patients and Families."
11. Refuse treatment and be told what effect this may have on your health.
12. Refuse to take part in research. In deciding whether or not to participate, you have the right to a full explanation.
13. Privacy while in the hospital and confidentiality of all information and records regarding your care.
14. Participate in all decisions about your treatment and discharge from the hospital. The hospital must provide you with a written discharge plan and written description of how you can appeal your discharge.
15. Review your medical record without charge and obtain a copy of your medical record for which the hospital can charge a reasonable fee. You cannot be denied a copy solely because you cannot afford to pay.
16. Complain without fear of reprisals about the care and services you are receiving and to have the hospital respond to you and if you request, a written response. If you are not satisfied with the hospital's response you can complain to the New York State Health Department. The hospital must provide you with the Health Department telephone number.

Items 8, 9, 11 and 12 are particularly relevant for patients with major illness, such as cancer or AIDS. These are:
Receive complete information about your diagnosis, treatment and prognosis.
Receive all the information you need to give informed consent for any proposed procedure or treatment. This information shall include the possible risks and benefits of the procedure or treatment.
Refuse to take part in research. In deciding where or not to participate, you have the right to a full explanation.

bined to prepare these graduates for responsible careers as genetic counselors. By 1993, increasing numbers of genetic counselors were specializing in the area of cancer genetic counseling.(3) A review of their training illustrates their appropriateness as cancer counselors.

The graduate program in Human Genetics at Sarah Lawrence College is an interdisciplinary two year program combining a medical genetics curriculum with training in counseling and patient advocacy. The two year curriculum for training non-physician genetic counselors is described below in Tables 2 and 3.

CURRICULUM FOR TRAINING NON-PHYSICIAN GENETIC COUNSELORS

The Medical Genetics course in year two includes nine hours of coursework in cancer genetics and cancer genetic counseling. A three hour lecture given by a prominent

Table 2. First year curriculum

Fall Semester	Spring Semester
Advanced Human Genetics	Human Physiology
Embryology	Biochemistry of Genetic Diseases
Biochemistry Review (1/2 semester)	Reproductive Genetics
Cytogenetics & Biochemical Labs	Issues in Genetic Counseling I
Issues in Genetic Counseling I	Introduction to Clinical Medicine (1/2 semester)
Client Centered Counseling Fieldwork (Lab)	Delivery of Genetic Services (1/4 semester)
	Journal Club
	Fieldwork (Counseling)

medical oncologist covers all issues of breast cancer diagnosis, treatment and predictive testing issues and implications. Most students in the program are exposed to cancer counseling under the supervision of certified genetic counselors in major cancer centers in the New York area.

The growth of consumerism in the delivery of medical services has seen a demand on the part of patients for active involvement in the management of their health care. This observation implies a subtle shifting of control from the doctor to the patient. When resources are limited, as they are in every country today, this balance of power become significant. However, empowering patients to advocate for themselves has been shown to have a positive effect psychologically in compliance with medical regimens. These factors can lead to a better quality of life, even for the most seriously ill patient. The literature strongly supports the connection between illness/poor quality of life, and loss of control. (4)

Cancer patients working with a genetic counselor advocate are helped in four ways:

1. To understand the diagnosis and how it was confirmed.
2. To review the genetic implication of the diagnosis for the patient and the family.
3. To understand the treatment regime or preventative action recommended by the physician.
4. To clarify the options available for care and their quality of life implications for the patient.
5. To have the opportunity to discuss the effect of the diagnosis on one's psychological well being.

Each of these activities supports the patient's confidence in their ability to understand the issues which, in turn, promotes the sense that they have gained some control over their life and are not at the mercy of the doctor and/or the hospital. Regaining this sense of autonomy can be important in helping patients to make their own health care de-

Table 3. Second year curriculum

Fall Semester	Spring Semester
Medical Genetics (two semesters)	Seminar in Genetic Counseling (two semesters)
Issues in Genetic Counseling (one semester)	Delivery of Genetic Services (1/2 semester)
Journal Club II	AIDS Workshop
Oral Examination	Cross Cultural Workshops (2)
Thesis	Fieldwork (Counseling)

cisions. Patients who feel in control are more likely to comply with recommended proce-dures.

PREDICTIVE TESTING

Inherited susceptibility to common adult onset cancers poses new opportunities for earlier treatment. The identification of individuals who may be at significant increased risk of developing malignant disease now include those with inherited colon, breast and ovarian cancer. Patients so identified will need to understand the associated risks for their families and that the results of their testing may identify family members who do not want to know their genetic status. The potential emotional component of gene testing is not anything patients should be expected to anticipate without the guidance of health profes-sionals. Non-carriers may also feel guilty that they have escaped (so called survivor guilt) (5).

COMPONENTS OF GENETIC COUNSELING

Genetic counseling must accompany genetic testing. Counseling must include:

1. Education: The patient/family must understand the genetics of their disease and the recommended treatment protocols.
2. Family History: Genetic counseling must include an exploration of specific is-sues related to the family history and experience with the condition they have. These experiences can span many generations and can include close personal in-volvement with relatives who have had cancer. Issues such as denial of disease risk or stigmatization of cancer within the family are important components of the history taking process. An understanding of the patients perspective is cru-cial.
3. Exploring Perception of Risk: The decision to undergo genetic testing should be made freely after careful consideration of the consequences of genetic testing. Exploration of the patient's views about risk and its meaning as well as the meaning of test results must be covered in a genetic session. The genetic coun-selor advocate must take responsibility for exploring these areas of cancer even when the patient appears reluctant to do so.
4. Disclosure of Test Results: Test results should be discussed in person with pa-tients and another review of the meaning and implications of the test under-taken. Follow-up sessions are often indicated to provide the patient with a second opportunity to ask additional questions and to assess whether further psychological support is needed. Issues of genetic discrimination in areas of in-surability or in the workplace may be appropriate to discuss at this time.(6)

SUMMARY

Having a genetic counseling professional as part of the oncology team can improve the care of patients, assist physicians in managing large patient populations and provide an important connection between the research goals of some oncology groups and patient needs. While our knowledge about cancer and cancer susceptibility in increasing rapidly, greater information needs to be generated about how best to deliver cancer information to the patient and family in the most constructive way.

REFERENCES

1. AHA (1973) Patient's Bill of Rights: American Hospital Association.
2. JCAHO (1994) Accreditation Material for Hospitals, Joint Commission for Accreditation of Health Care Organizations, Oakbrook Terrace, Chicago, Illinois.
3. Schneider KA. Counseling about Cancer. Strategies for Genetic Counselors. Dennisport, MA: Graphic Illusions, 1994.
4. Anderson BL. Psychological interventions for cancer patients to enhance the quality of life. Journal Consulting Clinical Psychology, 1992; 60:552–568.
5. Lerman C, Daly M, Masy A, et al. Attitudes about genetic testing for breast-ovarian cancer susceptibility. Journal of Clinical Oncology 1994; 12:843–850.
6. Carter MA. Patient provider relationship in the context of genetic testing for hereditary cancer. Monograph, National Cancer Institute 1995; 17:119–121.

13

RISK AS DIAGNOSIS

Implications for the Quality of Life

Lisbeth Sachs

Department of International Health and Social Medicine
IHCAR
Karolinska Institute
171 77 Stockholm, Sweden

INTRODUCTION

For an anthropologist it is a great challenge to discuss the concept Quality of Life in relation to health. In this paper I will present some of my thoughts on the subject that hopefully will provide ideas for fruitful discussion.

The Quality of Life for people in our part of the world is increasingly defined and created in health care situations where a complex set of cultural and social phenomena are involved. Health care has become the institution where we take our existential questions and where we seem to put much of our destiny and thoughts for future life and health. Because of the enormous expectations and hopes put on health care today and the power that comes with it, I argue that health care through advanced medical technology and diagnostic intruments not only saves lives but initiates suffering as well. Thus suffering occurs in people without symptoms, people who are not even detected as diseased. The suffering comes from the diagnosis of risk for future disease.

To be able to discuss this thesis I shall first take as an example how quality of life is defined within health care situations of a specific kind. The case is from a relatively new practice within health care in our Western world - the consultation service for genetic screening dealing with hereditary cancer.

While genetic screening is in a dynamic phase of development, with research presently being carried out in many parts of the developed world, counselling for 'cancer patients and families' is in its infancy in Sweden. Sweden is however now one of a limited number of countries with such clinical application of genetic research. Genetic screening is not, at this point, utilized for general populations, but its use in Stockholm is limited to those persons who are believed or believe themselves to be at risk for hereditary cancer. It is relatively new and unfamiliar to both health care providers and laypersons.

Cancer, AIDS, and Quality of Life, edited by Levy *et al.*
Plenum Press, New York, 1997

I have worked with a research project concerning the consultation service for genetic screening which is presently in existence at the Department of Genetics, at The Karolinska Institute in Stockholm. Two physicians with backgrounds in clinical genetics, surgery and oncology are engaged in this new program. 'Patients' come to this clinic through direct contact, referrals by other physicians, or contact mediated by family members who have either a cancer diagnosis, or a hereditary risk. A physician meets with the patients, a genogram is drawn up to chart hereditary factors and counselling on individual risk and preventive alternatives are provided. Breast, cervix and colorectal cancer are the hereditary syndromes most commonly presented, but people with questions concerning other cancer forms are also seen at the consultation service. The mere opportunity given as to possible risk for future disease makes people eager to know their own 'destiny'.

The general aim of the study was to describe the process whereby persons experiencing themselves as 'well' come to perceive risk, or not, in connection with cancer prevention, and to describe how this experience is dealt with and made sense of by the involved participants, both professionals and the potential patient (1).

The determination of risk status of an individual for development of a cancer is a complex process, involving negotiations between different modes of discussion (2). There is risk on the scientific dimension, expressed in objective terms, derived from the population-based study of epidemiology or genetic research. There is also a dimension of risk, as experienced both by health care practitioners and the individual 'potential patient'.

At least two processes of translation are involved in the conversion of data from the biomedical research on risk (Figure 1). These include the statistics derived from population-based studies that are to be translated into clinical knowledge and practice. They have to be put into a language of risk which can communicate the risk- diagnosis into the lay world of interpretation and understanding.

The mere information about risk for a deadly disease leads to consequences for the women with a genogram showing a picture of, for example, hereditary breast cancer. How do they understand their own risk? In the project we have recorded and transcribed 30 information talks between the clinician and the 'patient'. Ten of these patients have now been followed for two years during which time half of them have gone through prophylactic operations while the others are still in the process of deciding.

THE LANGUAGE OF RISK

The practitioners who engage in preventive information are enmeshed in the dilemmas of medical uncertainty about what is known and what is unknown about the future of possible disease. The concept of risk plays a central role in understandings about the etiology and prevention of chronic disease both in epidemiology and in clinical medicine. When translated into clinical practice and lay perceptions, however, the concept becomes

Statistical level

Clinical knowledge and practice

An individual life situation

Figure 1. Levels of translation.

more broadly defined (3). Within clinical and lay contexts it is more appropriate to speak of *the language of risk* in that the term is used to convey a constellation of meanings some of which are intended and some of which remain largely unconscious (4). The language of risk is about scientific uncertainty concerning causal relationships, and clinical and lay uncertainty concerning the prediction and control of unhealthy outcomes. And how is the concept of risk perceived and made sense of in the personal life of each of these women?

RISK AS DIAGNOSIS

The search for personal control over risk often leads to further medical approaches. Because the women feel helpless to do anything to change their risk on their own, they are left at the hands of medical experts. The data in this study suggest that while it is clear that the women do not have cancer, they are diagosed with a risk for cancer which means that they are in some sense given a sickness (2). This information causes the women to be uncertain if they should consider themselves healthy or ill. The women feel that they have no alternatives but to continue with medical surveillance or prophylactic removal of their breasts. Faced with the fear of breast cancer as a possible outcome, knowing that there is no way to prevent the disease but to do a prophylactic operation, the women are healthy but have a diagnosis of risk which they have to consider. In their current state the women are not in a position to walk away from the knowledge that they have been given. In a very real sense, being diagnosed at risk is itself a risk factor and an invisible cause to a personal dilemma which leads to implications for their future lives.

THE CONCEPT OF HEALTH

Here I need to introduce a theoretical consideration about the concept of health to be able to follow through my argument. Quality of Life is inherent in what we mean by health. But the concept of health may be just as difficult to define as is the concept of Quality of Life. They both are individual and social, personal and cultural.

The changing norms related to health and sickness in our modern Western world, in combination with the use of highly developed diagnostic techniques, create a situation in which a cancer diagnosis may now be determined without any 'illness' on the part of the potential patient, but through screening procedures which discover potential 'disease' (5). Here I want to define the concepts of illness and disease more in detail since they are central to my argument.

Illness comprises expressions for the subjective perceptions (symptoms) which are not necessarily visible (pain) but are communicated, verbally or otherwise, in a culturally prescribed manner.

The direct observations which a physician can make in encounters with patients whose language and means of expression he or she understands, are manifestations of illness in the sense used here.

The physician may also discover signs of which the patient is unaware (e.g. fever, anemia, elevated blood pressure, cellular changes, HIV infections). The physician can do this even without understanding the patient's language or means of expression. He does not even need the patients active assistance.

Disease is a state of ill-health (not necessarily perceived) arising from an objective pathology, mainly obtained through medical technology, and classified, explained and treated in biomedical terms.

In order to claim that illness is caused by biological changes - that disease is present - one therefore needs objective evidence of what is going on in the body. It is only specialists in the scientific sector who can obtain such evidence, above all by using medical technology.

When a physician cannot establish a diagnosis that matches the patient´s symptoms, the illness for which the patient has applied for help, one can say that illness is present without detectable disease. In other cases it is illness which prompts the physician to detect the disease, and then they are both present. These two situations often automatically lead to an unhealthy feeling and some kind of suffering.

Besides confirming illness as a disease we have in our health care in the West an *active search* for disease without illness. If we go outside of Sweden and the Western world, however, we may discover that most people are not accustomed to health check-ups or preventive health care of this kind. Curative care is the main occupation in developing countries. For many it is not relevant to examine the body beneath its surface especially if the person is healthy. Ill health is only what is felt and observed as a changed state in an individual member of the group or society.

Let us look at the definition of Health made by WHO and see how it fits with this model of health and ill-health and what it has to say about the Quality of Life.

Health is a state of complete physical, mental, and social well-being and not merely the absence of disease or infirmity.

And the revised definition:

Health is a state of physical, mental, and social wellbeing with or without disease or infirmity.

This revised definition takes into account people in a global perspective who are not screened for an asymptomatic, invisible disease but feel healthy. To feel healthy, to have a good quality of life may also include people with various chronic diseases and handicaps.

The normal state for most people in the non-Western world is the notion that what is not felt or what is not visible does not result in suffering. We may however need a third definition since for us in the Western world what is not visible is also haunting us and gives us suffering. The mere possibility today to visualize the invisible and to give prognostic invisible risk- profiles create a situation much more complex than we are able to grasp. So if we attempt to discuss the definitions of Quality of Life in relation to health, a third concept besides illness and disease would be appropriate and fruitful. The concept is sickness (6).

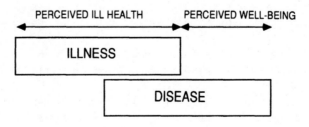

Figure 2. The relationship between illness and disease.

Sickness is a socially important state, a sick-role, more or less unrelated to whether there is defined illness or disease or both. Un-health is not a socially important phenomenon until it is recognised by others. The person who is given a sick-role enters a role with altered rights and responsibilities.

In any society, illness must be read and understood by the other members to be legitimized as sickness. People in society who have this authority may be regarded as gate-keepers. Gate-keepers must name the ailment, and by doing that confirm that the person in question is sick. Some kind of treatment can be given once the ailment is named and confirmed. But the most important is that the sick-role is legitimized. This fact also means that the person enters a social role when he or she can refrain from responsibilities in everyday life.

The message here then is that sickness is a useful concept if we want to talk about Quality of Life and health in a cultural context. We need a concept that will help us put a focus on society and culture as the structures where male and female sick roles are created and recreated, accepted or refused. Society uses deviance as a structuring device and sickness is one of them. Let us try to investigate how this is done in this process. Any understanding of the impact of health problems in the future must in my view take into consideration, the issues that focus on sickness and the gate-keeper's authority to legitimize this state.

While disease is the central concern in therapeutic encounters with medical care, and illness is the central concern from the standpoint of the affected individual, it is sickness that is of central importance in understanding social behavior. It is the social definition that triggers contact with gate-keepers like health professionals and that orders social participation. A question which remains as yet unexplored but appears particularly salient then, is the relationship of sickness to the screening process. It can be postulated that programs for secondary prevention and screening provide socially significant meanings and significant outcomes without the existence of either disease or illness. Is it possible that the screening process itself may lead to "sickness" experience?

The relationship between illness-disease-sickness-and-risk is presented in Fig. 3.

Let me come back to the women who are given risk as a diagnosis and look at the concept of sickness in relation to themselves. Sickness is in this description not something to be observed. It is an invisible and implicit state of suffering that has been introduced in the women's lives through a practice which still has a lot of medical uncertainty and risk in itself.

Risk becomes both a symptom of future disease and a current sickness; a perception of ill-health.

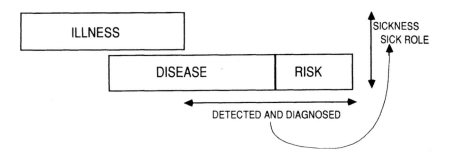

Figure 3. The relationship between illness-disease-sickness-risk.

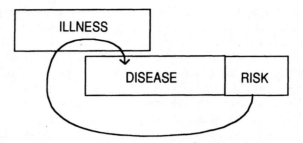

Figure 4. The relationship between risk and illness/disease.

When the women choose to resolve the conflict through the removal of their breasts or ovaries, a new situation occured. While the practitioners were successful in gaining control over a physical condition, the women suffered from the removal of part of their bodies. Thus while doctors can deal with risk through surgery, the women get their risks transformed into a new physical state of ill-health.

As the women whom I have followed for two years now, have gotten their risk articulated their lives have become totally changed. Those who have made the decision to have an operation have to go through all the pain and adaptation to the new body. They continue to suffer from thoughts that the operation has perhaps not been totally sucessful, or that the cancer may come in some other part of the body. They do not necessarily continue their lives with the feeling that they have been 'cured'. They go on living with their identity as risk-persons in a state of sickness.

My argument is that the overall health as essential for the Quality of life is defined at various levels at the same time within each health care situation dealing with the invisible risks for future disease. All is related in a complex way which is difficult to foresee. Each person within a screening program has a specific way of dealing with bad news in his or her personal lifesituation. It is not possible ahead of time to make a prognosis of how the screening will introduce a lifelong suffering to an individual.

The relationship between risk and illness/disease is presented in Figure 4.

As an anthropologist I am interested in how life experiences and feelings such as fear, joy, mourning, end euphoria, build the base for health or un-health (7). The question that I want to pose is whether these women who are *well* but get a risk diagnosis for future disease will be able to stay healthy if they start suffering from anxiety and fear. What are the experiences and feelings that will trigger pathological processes? In the new psychoneuroimmunological research the message is that feelings do kill and feelings can heal. Before there are means to treat all that is possible to discover through genetic screening, the diagnosis of risk may mean more harm than relief. What does constant anxiety lead to? What does the Quality of life have to do with health? Do we in the Western world undermine the Quality of life for people through our search for the invisible health risks? There are more questions than answers.

May we venture to say that Quality of life is:

A state of physical, mental, and social wellbeing with or without disease or infirmity or the awareness of disease and future risks?

ACKNOWLEDGMENT

The study referred to in this presentation was made possible through a generous grant from the Swedish Council for Planning and Coordination of Research.

REFERENCES

1. Sachs, L. and Tishelman, C. Between Sickness and Health, an interdisciplinary exploration of secondary prevention of cancer and the fluctuating meaning of health.(Unpublished research proposal) 1993.
2. Gifford, S.M.The meaning of lumps: a case study of the ambiguities of risk. In C.R. Janes et al eds. Anthropology and Epidemiology, D.Reidel Publishing Co pp 1986;213–246.
3. Rose, G. Sick individuals and sick populations. International Journal of Epidemiology 1985;14:32–38.
4. Adelswärd, V. and Sachs, L. The meaning of 6,8 : numeracy and normality in health information talks. Social Science and Medicine (in press) 1996.
5. Kleinman, A., Eisenberg, L. and Good, B. Culture, illness and care: clinical lessons from anthropologic and cross-cultural research. Annals Intern. Med.1978;88:251–258.
6. Young, A. The anthropologies of illness and sickness. Ann. Rev. Anthropol.1982;257–285.
7. Sachs, L. Is there a pathology of prevention? The implications of visualizing the invisible in screening programs. Culture, Medicine and Psychiatry, 1995;19:503–525.

14

QUALITY OF LIFE AS A MAJOR DETERMINANT OF MEDICAL DECISION-MAKING

Robert Zittoun

Service d'Hématologie
Hôtel-Dieu
1, place du Parvis Notre Dame
75181 Paris Cedex 04, France

In this paper, I shall mainly consider the second part of the question: Not so much who defines quality of life; we know that it has been or can be done by several categories: philosophers, social scientists, physicians, companies (especially pharmaceutical companies), health administration, government ... But rather who makes medical-decisions and how determination of quality of life and other determinants may contribute to a medical decision (1). Medical decisions are mainly made by physicians, but through quality of life or other determinants, the other categories contribute to this decision.

In fact, as already said, there are hundreds of definitions of quality of life, which normally include several dimensions of life, with, in addition, different weights from one individual to the other, from time to time, By contrast, there is only one medical-decision at a given time, followed eventually by secondary decisions on consecutive times, whatever be the value judgement which underlines this decision and its degree of uncertainty.

Another point must be emphasized: there is an increasing demand of cancer and AIDS patients for information and participation in medical decision-making. This trend is observed in many different countries, with varied cultural backgrounds, all over the world, and is related to the shift from paternalism to personalism in the patient-physician relationship.

Nowadays, most treatment choices are conditioned by guidelines or constraints from health administration. We observe an increasing role of clinical trials evaluating the various treatment strategies. To consolidate and rationalize the bases of the decision, overviews, meta-analyses and consensus conferences are rapidly growing. Furthermore, the ethical aspects are also homogenized throughout countries and cultures, not only for inclusion in clinical trials, but also for acceptance of an individual decision outside such trials. The role of proxies in case of patient's incompetence has been defined as well

This consensual approach of medical decision-making raises, however, a series of medical, anthropological and ethical questions:

Cancer, AIDS, and Quality of Life, edited by Levy *et al.*
Plenum Press, New York, 1997

- Too frequently, these methods oriented towards a consensual decision have resulted in a corpus of ideologically dominant practices, that the patient is invited to adopt regardless of his/her individual values and preferences.
- Such practice may lead to return to an insidiously paternalistic model, where physicians, specialists, companies and health-policy deciders dictate the "best" choice. The patient is just asked to provide a formal "informed consent".
- Some modern medical behaviours, related to protocols and clinial trials, are just scandalous and should be more clearly denounced, and the perverse effects of the present ethical regulations should be analyzed.

Yet, the premises of an alternative model do exist. The ways of eliciting a patient, individual values and preferences have been worked through and illustrated, despite methodological difficulties (2). This objective can be achieved especially for several critical choices where patients individual preferences should be incorporated. For example, choosing:

- between different levels of iatrogenic morbidity and mortality, which corresponds to risk acceptance
- or between different ways to control the disease, which results in differences in remission duration, survival, and quality of life. The integration of quality of life and survival duration results in quality-adjusted life years (so-called QALY) (3). Here, it is not so much the QALYs calculated by the insurance companies, but rather the quality-adjusted life expectancy, according to the patient wishes.

Major fields should be identified where critical decisions have frequently to be made. In my experience, as a clinician involved in hemato-oncology, such criticial situations are frequently observed in the treatment of leukemias. For example:

- Performing or not a bone marrow transplant, a high risk procedure, at the beginning of a chronic and otherwise uncurable leukemia.
- At a later phase, adopting a palliative treatment, or, on the contrary, proposing to the patient to enter a phase I/II clinical trial.
- Also adopting a Do-Not-Ressucitate procedure, according to the chances of cure and to the patient's advance requests.

To illustrate the first point, I would like to summarize the results of a clinical trial performed by our European EORTC Cooperative Group in patients with acute myelogenous leukemia during first remission (4). About one thousand patients were incorporated in this study from 1986 to 1992. Three treatments, allogeneic bone marrow transplantation (AlloBMT), autologous bone marrow transplantation (ABMT) and intensive chemotherapy consolidation were allocated by genetic chance or central randomization (IC).

AlloBMT results in a lower relapse risk, than ABMT, then IC. But, with regards to the treatment-related mortality, the results were the opposite: 20 % for alloBMT, 10 % for ABMT and 5 % for IC. AlloBMT and ABMT resulted in an equivalent disease-free survival, significantly longer than IC. However the overall survival was equivalent for the three arms: the patients in the IC arm were more easily salvaged after relapse, with secondary ABMT. We analyzed afterwards the quality of life of patients during long-term remission, 1 to 8 years after completion of treatment. We used the EORTC Core questionnaire, plus specific modules for leukemia, for infertility and sexuality, and for perceived changes by the patient as compared to the pre-disease state. The results, recently presented (5), indicated that AlloBMT results is lower overall and specific values of quality of life, especially with regards to infertility, which is permanent, and sexuality. Then comes ABMT, and the best figures are given by patients treated in the IC arm. Other comparisons have to be made, especially with regard to cost-effectiveness. The first indication gives alloBMT as the most expansive, then ABMT, then IC.

The conclusion to be drawn from this study is that there is no one magic criteria or a best choice. I think that risk factors and patient preferences should be incoporated, which can be done even in the future clinical trials as stratification or exclusions factors. Weighting and incorporating patient preferences and values, with regard to life expectancy and quality of life should be a major field of medical research and education.

REFERENCES

1. Moinpour CM., Feigl P., Metch B., Hayden KA., Meyskens FL., Crowley J.: Quality of life end points in cancer clinical trials: review and recommendations. Journal of the National Cancer Institute. 1989, 81: 485–495.
2. O'Connor AMC., Boyd NF., Warde P., Stolbach L., Till JE: Eliciting preferences for alternative drug therapies in oncology: influence of treatment outcome description, elicitation tehcnique and treatment experience on preferences. Journal of Chronic Diseases. 1985, 40: 811–815.
3. Torrance GW., Feeny D.: Utilities and quality-adjusted life years. International Journal of Technology Assessment in Health Care. 1989, 5: 559–575.
4. Zittoun R., Mandelli F., Willemze R et al. Autologous or allogeneic bone marrow transplantation compared with intensive chemotherapy in acute myelogenous leukemia. New England Journal of Medicine 1995, 332: 217–223.
5. Zittoun R., Suciu S., Solbu G et al. Comparison of quality of life (QOL) of patients with acute myelogenous leukemias (AML) in long-term first complete remission (CR) after bone marrow transplantation (BMT) - allogeneic or autologous - or intensive chemotherapy consolidation (ICC): EORTC-GIMEMA AML 8 A study. Blood 1995, 86, supp'.1: 433a.

15

QUALITY OF LIFE AT THE END STAGES OF LIFE

Mohammed Bedjaoui

Court Internationale de Justice
Palais de la Paix
NL-2517 KJ la Haye
Pays-Bas

I. THE CONCEPT OF QUALITY OF LIFE

Subjective and Objective Aspects

Quality of life is above all *a subjective concept* and thus variable according to the individual, but at the same time sensitive to the environment in which we live. Quality of life is, in the first place, like the proverbial Spanish inn, where the visitor only finds what he has brought along himself. It is a manner of being, a manner of feeling, a way of *appreciating* life (in the etymological sense of the verb, i.e., ascribing its *true value* to life, whether high or - on the contrary - insignificant, according to one's current state of mind). That *appreciation* is particularly subjective. It is the *private domain* of each individual. That quality of life is also the art of being able to create all the conditions needed to make a success of *one's* own life or, more precisely, what one sees oneself as constituting success.

That *quality of life* depends on a large number of factors to *"make a life"* for oneself or to achieve *"self-fulfilment"*. It depends on *physical* aptitudes (it is no use dreaming of becoming a great footballer if one has a heart condition). It is conditioned by *intellectual* aptitudes (not everyone can be a professor or research scientist). It depends upon certain gifts (not everyone can be a musician or painter, or a star of stage or screen). However, it also depends upon a person's *social environment*, *economic* circumstances or even *entourage*, as well as on the *character of the person* concerned (i.e., whether they are ambitious or self-effacing).

That quality of life will above all vary according to the *options* that one effects, i.e.,

- the choice of an *occupation* (exciting or frustrating)
- the choice of a *spouse* (the companion of a lifetime)
- the choice of *hobbies or pastimes* (which give expression to a taste for taking risks or a search for relaxation in secure surroundings and the elevation of one's spirit)
- the choice of *friends*, the choice of relationships including one's relationship with one's own secretary . . .
- even the choice of *food* has its significance.

As you know, the *multinational* companies that produce all sorts of things in order to improve - according to them - our quality of life, to make things easier for the housewife, etc., have only one real objective, that of extending their markets on a global scale. It follows that those multinationals *condition* us in our *tastes*, shape us in our *options* in favour of certain kinds of food and clothing or in our leisure time activities, and in everything that contributes to the quality of life. They impose upon us fast-food restaurants, coca cola, jazz or blue denim, as well as certain types of classical music or holidays. We make our choices to improve our quality of life, but *in fact* they condition us, totally or almost totally, in those choices.

However the quality of life remains an essentially personal problem.

- It depends upon individuals: this is the *personal factor*: *"What would be an acceptable way of ending one's life"*? The answers differ from one person to another;
- it depends upon the length of expectation of life or the length of the respite afforded to a sick person: it is the *time factor*, or the familiar question: *"If you only had thirty minutes to life, what would you want to do?";*
- it also depends upon *financial means* and *opportunities*. Jacques Brel went to end his short life in Tahiti. François Mitterand went off to admire eternity in the civilization of Lower Egypt, and then chose the day of his death;
- it depends upon *religious factors*. Some religions are more fatalistic, more resigned than others. Some even prefer to the sad life on earth, which is no more than a vale of tears, the life hereafter with its rewards of bliss;
- it depends upon age. A child is entirely happy if he has his favourite toy or his mother's caressing smile; the adolescent aspires to explore even further the richness of life; the adult has other expectations and the old man other kinds of anguish;
- lastly, it depends upon the way in which one copes with the transition from active life to *retirement*. One general was able to explain his difficulties in adapting to retirement in a restaurant, when he exclaimed *"to say that I have been reduced to ordering a dish of sauerkraut after having given orders to a regiment for so long!"*

However all the different parameters which condition or fashion the quality of a human life do not mean that there is no room for personal intervention. *One forges one's own happiness to a fairly large extent.* A keen gardener who manages to grow a magnificent plant from a cutting or who lovingly gazes upon the roses or petunias that he has himself planted and tended, is giving himself a certain quality of life, essentially brought about by his own efforts.

Some authors dream of the creation of a *science of the quality* of life. This would be aimed at suggesting actions such as to improve the quality of life, promoting the best possible options, guaranteeing the necessary facilities, directing efforts towards useful actions by assisting in their structuring and by coordinating them in such a way as to ensure that the quality of life meets current requirements or responds to current wishes - requirements and wishes of society as much as of the individual, the former being aimed at an improved distribution of material resources or, in other words, working on a policy of *quantity* the better to insure the *quality* of life for all, and the latter relating to the subjective perception of that quality and the attainment of personal objectives.

How can one characterise the sequence being examined by our symposium? The end stages that we are studying constitute the phase of palliative care, *the phase in which the quality of life must be the most demanding, but when in fact only the most mediocre standard is assured, by force of circumstance.* This is the phase in which all the protagonists, including the sick person, know and acknowledge that nothing more can be done. It is the phase of powerlessness. This is tragic for the patient, but is also tragic for those taking care of him, to a certain extent. Protocol can no longer be applied. The possibilities of a cure - if there ever were any - have definitively ceased to exist.

It is, then, qualitatively another phase; an new relationship between the patient and those looking after him. It is a great deal more demanding, as the patient wants more *comfort* than ever at a time at which, on the one hand, his aggravated physical degeneration makes this less of an option and when, moreover, curative treatment can no longer be given and when nothing more than inevitably limited palliative treatment is available. In these circumstances, *dependency is evidence of a severance of relations*, a severance that is unbearable for all concerned, for both patients and those taking care of them.

II. THE PHYSICIAN, THE LAWYER AND THE MORALIST CONFRONTED BY THE QUESTION OF THE QUALITY OF THE END STAGES OF LIFE

Not long since, just a few decades ago, the blueprint of the relations between the patient and the physician was fairly clear, and a watching brief was kept by lawyers, legislators and philosophers. The practitioner - as he was called - and his patient entered into and maintained a controlled relationship, without any major risks and without any great surprises. Today, on the contrary, the scene has changed. The curtain goes up to reveal an unfamiliar set. The protagonists - the physician and the patient - are joined by the legislator who has hastened to catch up on events, by the philosopher intervening to reconcile science and conscience, by the lawyer alert to the need to harmonize different interests in good order and legality. All those actors are required to perform in a difficult play, without any false notes or hidden prompter and without fumbling their lines. It is a play without hope, without any possible happy ending, as the powerless physician capitulates and sadly signs the statement "The End" - in all the possible meanings of that term.

This play is about the *departure* of a man, an inevitable departure, which must not even be delayed any further. Aggressive care has no meaning in that context. There is nothing more to hope for given the onslaught of cancer, of aids, which threatens mankind. One must only attempt to accompany the patient on his final voyage, in the most dignified manner.

Organizing palliative care, providing support for the dying person, humanizing the last phases of his life. To that end, the scenes that must be impeccably played out in this drama with no happy ending, are called *changes in the nature of medicine*, the *free choice* and *consent of the patient*, the *responsibility* and *solidarity of all concerned* and, in particular, the medical personnel and the family.

A. Changes in the Nature of Medicine

In the old days, the physician relieved symptoms, repaired damage and extended life when he could, as well as assisting the sick person. He continues to do so, of course, but *medicine has already, before our eyes, changed its function and even its nature*. With genetic engineering and the biological sciences, it now has the power to modify, improve or tamper with the processes of a living person.

We are becoming involved in a kind of medicine which responds not only to *suffering*, but also to *needs* and which is capable of meeting those needs, such as the *"desire for a child"* of a childless couple or a woman on her own, thanks to the progress of genetic techniques and medically assisted procreation. This means that medicine has opened up to the *quality of life*, that it is freeing hopes, building happiness and forging new human rights.

In short, medicine, which has changed before our eyes, does not confine its ambitions to providing health care and extending life (the *"quantity of life"* objective), but also aims to contribute to the provision of a *"quality of life"*. Nothing is more striking than the current proliferation of medication to promote well-being and "happiness pills". Physicians have long been aware of the fact that quality of life is not only a *state of health*, but also a *state of mind*, as Dr. Feinstein said.

Among the new human rights are included *the rights of the sick person* whose unspeakable sufferings have to be assuaged when he cannot be freed of them, and who must be accompanied in his last days by palliative care imbued with humanity.

The world of medicine is undergoing a change. However, in a number of respects, our *legal system of reference* is not yet able to provide a framework for these new acts of the physician, who is now concerned with the quality *of the end stages* of life. *This new medicine is waiting for a new legality with appropriate ethical markers*. Medicine has not left it to the more or less fortunate inspiration of one of its own experts to effect the ethical choices implied by certain acts at the end of a life. Ever since Hippocrates, medicine has provided itself with a code of ethics. In ancient times or in the middle ages, the physician was often reinforced by the philosopher. Fortunately, this is still frequently the case today. Today he is starting to *listen to the patient*, who teaches him a great deal. He is starting to listen to public opinion, and to ethical committees which have increased in number. He is thus regaining contact with the need to take account of the *whole man* and not of the *disjointed man*, broken down into his separate parts.

One needs to define, with renewed attention, the *eminently strategic place of the physician* in society, if society is not to lose its humanity in the face of death.

B. The Consent of the Patient

For an acceptable quality of life at the end stages, an essential requirement is the consent of the patient to all the significant initiatives that the physician must take. After all, one is talking about his life and his end. Questions relating to the information of the patient as to his real state of health, *"aggressive care"*, the duration of palliative care and its limitations, euthanasia in those countries where it has been legalized, etc . . ., cannot be conceived without the appropriate intervention of the patient's consent.

The Patient's "Living Will".
In order to keep their status as human beings, people must help each other not to lose their *eminent dignity*. However *"human dignity"* is an apparently simple expression of which one can immediately grasp, if not the precise meaning, at least the scope in perspective. But it is also, paradoxically, an expression laden with fragilities, as some people use the same argument of *"human dignity"* to refute the *legitimacy of euthanasia* while others claim this to be the ultimate right of whosoever intends to *"die in dignity"!* It is difficult to act with all the requisite discernment in the final phase of life, in order to assist the person who is dying.

Today, men and women, moved by a concern for their dignity as they understand it, draw up what are known as *"living wills"*, or, in other words, declarations of intent to die in *"dignity"*, rejecting in advance the concept of "aggressive care", physical or mental decay, hopeless suffering and a degrading dependence upon others. Thus we have in circulation various manifestoes aimed at promoting *"easy death"* - a sign of the times.

A Human Contract Based on Truth and Trust.
One of the delicate issues that arises during this *"voyage to the end of life"* is that of whether the doctor should tell the patient everything about his state and let him know *approximately how long he still has to live.* This is the *"Crónica de una muerte anunciada"*.

Look at what happened in the two films by Mr. Cavada, that were shown yesterday afternoon. The old gentlemen knew his death was scheduled for the near future. He went through that phase of palliative care *in the light of that truth that was so hard to bear.* After all, when a patient is in a *palliative care* unit, he is bound to hypothesize that a definitive corner has been turned and that there is no more room for *curative measures*.

Now think, if you will, of Mr. Cavada's second film. That woman who was so very much alive knew that she was *condemned in the short term* but, unlike the gentleman in the first film, did not believe - could not believe - that her end was so very close at hand. She described the diagnosis as *"science fiction"*. It is true that she was not in a palliative care unit.

The two films resemble each other in that each of those two people had learned of their approaching end from their doctor, but they differed from each other in that one believed in his diagnosis while the other did not believe in hers.

How should one reveal and how should one receive the truth, given this concern for the quality of life? Doubtless the relationship between doctor and patient may be analyzed in terms of a contract, a contract of trust, implying a relationship of truth. However this whole field seems to me to be a *matter of circumstances* and particular cases, as one is thinking of the quality of life and the final phase. The physician has to *feel*, on a case by case basis, whether it is a good idea to tell a patient the truth, given the concern for the quality of the end stages of life. In that regard, a great deal depends upon the patients themselves, as some would wish to know and others not.

In his dealings with patients the physician frequently learns a great deal himself. As was said at greater length by Marie de Hennezel in her book *"La mort intime"* ["Death on Intimate Terms"], "those who are going to die teach us to live". They can, among other things, guide the physician in his *duty to tell or to keep silent*.

The Wish for Death as a Deliverance from an Abominable Quality of the End Stages of Life.

The problem that arises in relation to the quality of the end stages of life, and which is even central to that question, is to know if and how the physician may cope with the entreaties of the patient who, invoking that quality of the end stages of life, desires that the doctor should help him to *die on a certain day of his own choice*.

I come from a country where I live, i.e. the Netherlands, in which *euthanasia* is legally acceptable. However the palliative care unit is not a place where you "go to die"; it is not an elephants' cemetery into which they withdraw with solemnity, and even with a certain dignity, placing themselves of their own accord outside the animal society of their group. In euthanasia, the doctor plays an active part as adviser, guide and executant. In the situation envisaged here it is, on the contrary, the patient who asks the doctor for death.

However the two situations are not that clear-cut. Situations of euthanasia arise, in places where it has not been legalized. The dialogue between the patient and the doctor is sometimes so *ambiguous by necessity* that there is no obvious difference between a situation of legalized euthanasia and an act of euthanasia in which the patient, his family and his doctor have collaborated in various ways.

I referred just now to the question of *"living wills"*. I shall not revert to it.

C. Solidarity and Responsibility

In the search for quality of life at the end stages of life, it is the indissociable binomial of solidarity and responsibility which will govern the final phase of the patient's existence.

One must generously mete out gestures of solidarity with sick people who are leaving on their last journey. Solidarity is something which tends to get lost in individualistic modern societies, which are as cold as steel. In that regard, *Africa*, of which *Professor Peter Piot* has graphically described the advanced state of physical dilapidation, at least possesses in its misfortune some admirable *traditions of solidarity*. Listen to this dialogue taken from the initiation ceremony of a young Mandingo:

"Who are you?"

"I am earth and water, plus something that I have to preserve, something that links me to the people of yesterday, today and tomorrow."

"Who are you?"

"I am nothing without you, I am nothing without them. When I came into the world, I was in their hands; they were there to welcome me. When I leave, I shall be in their hands; they will be there to accompany me to my last resting place".

In palliative care, *the struggle against pain becomes an essential factor in the quality of life at the end stages*. The right not to have to endure unspeakable agony becomes *one of the large number of human rights of patients in the terminal phase* and may lead to the alternative of euthanasia. Likewise, for the doctor, to dispense comfort remains *the only task still within his reach*, when he realises that his curative efforts are useless. Anaesthetists become *"doctors of pain"* to use the term employed by Dr. Michèle Salamagne.

When hope grows slender, when the light grows dim in the lamp of life, there is almost nothing else one can do than to continue to safeguard the *quality of life at the end stages*, which can essentially be summed up as a struggle against unspeakable agony. What can be done at that stage, is on the one hand to develop a mastery of *"therapeutic measures to provide comfort"* (it appears that we now have apparatus to make precise measurements of the quantities of morphine or other analgesics that are needed to cope with different intensities of pain); and also to develop the dying person's emotional environment in relation to his family.

When the pressure of pain attains an unbearable degree of tyranny, the whole of the palliative care unit is made to suffer, as the patient under the onslaught of pain will become aggressive himself. *The covenant between the patient, the physician and the family is broken*. One is tempted not to see the patient again. Then comes the time to administer lytic *"cocktails"* to put the patient to sleep, or, in other words, to ensure that one will not have to listen to him and that he will not hear himself crying out. Those "cocktails" constitute the *worst type of abdication*. However what can one do where there is no desire for euthanasia or where the patient himself has left no *"living will"*?

Yet another problem arises. *Medically, psychologically, emotionally* and *economically*, does the patient at the end stage need to go into a palliative care unit or to go back *to die among his own, surrounded by his own, with his own*? The situation is the following:

The doctor can do no more from a *curative* standpoint. Palliative care is *expensive* for the State or the patient. The patient needs the affection and the warmth of his family, and vice versa. I believe that, out of respect for this *quality of life at the end stages* and the expressed desire of by the patient and/or his family, he must be allowed to pass away within his family setting.

Pain, at *the end of life*, becomes what the British and Dr. Michèle Salamagne refer to as *"total agony"* in which there is virtually no quality of life at the end stages. The patient experiences unspeakable physical suffering, to which is however added a psychological agony or anguish, a feeling of isolation or even of rejection, a spiritual void. Discomfort is at its maximum. The *quality of life at the end stages* becomes an empty form of words.

III. WHAT CONCLUSIONS CAN WE DRAW?

(i) The challenges occasioned by someone who is dying are not only addressed to doctors, but also to lawyers, moralists and legislators. One may consider that the key to all the problems relating to the complex relationship between the physician, the patient and his family lies in the concept of *respect for the dignity* of the patient under all circumstances.

(ii) *New rights are coming into existence.* Human rights are being enriched by new conceptual advances. After the Charter of the Rights of the Child, the *rights of the patient* are taking shape. We are not talking about the patient with injuries occasioned on the battlefield who has been protected by the law of armed conflict and humanitarian law ever since the declaration of St. Petersbourg of 1868. We are talking of the *civilian patient*. The right to health is not in question: that right has long been recognized by various Constitutions throughout the world. The new right to which I refer is indeed a right to health for a patient who, after having been duly informed of the possibilities, might have a choice of treatments at each phase, and who wishes to get well without suffering or to die without discomfort.

A new blueprint for patients' rights is taking shape through the patient's free choice and informed consent, when confronted with the treatment proposed or the indications suggested. In short, at present, *the quality of care is directly linked to the quality of life, whereas it was previously linked to the attainment of a cure.*

(iii) *Do we need a science to complement medical science, which would be a science of quality?* Such a science would suggest the *requisite actions*, help to bring about a *choice of the best options*, guarantee the necessary facilities and, coordinate actions to ensure that the quality of life and the quality of the *end stages* of life would meet requirements. The experiment now under way will give an answer to this question.

(iv) However, when the patient embarks on his heroic final course, a problem arises of how all the protagonists should conduct themselves when confronted by incipient physical deterioration, the imminent triumph of death, developing agony, and so many factors which constitute a cruel challenge to the *quality of life at the end stages.* I do not think there is any *ready-made recipe* to be followed in all cases by each one of the actors in this moving drama.

There does not exist - there cannot exist, there must not exist - a sort of *Handbook* in twelve lessons to teach one how to help a patient at the end stage. The patient is asking for a very great deal, and the response of those caring for him is inevitably limited, in time, in resources and availability. There is no Guide or Handbook for the quality of life at the end stages. Patients and those taking care of them all have to learn how to cope, how to cope with that hard reality in which the one who gives the most is perhaps the patient himself. One *never stops* learning how to accompany *those who are dying*.

(v) The physician does not only cure, repair, assuage suffering and extend life; his ambition is to dispense more than wellbeing, almost *happiness*. The gestures of the physician and his indications, his prescriptions and his advice now also take account of the patient's comfort and wellbeing, especially when one is dealing with severe illnesses like cancer or aids, for which it seems all the more important to try to dispense wellbeing in that (1) treatments are themselves an ordeal and (2) their success is too limited to be able to obscure the hideous face of death which becomes the patient's close companion.

(vi) Within the framework of patients' rights there is, more especially, one right - the right *not to* know. That right ought to be protected, above all in the realm of predictive medicine. A person does not need to know that he possesses a gene which will, forty or fifty years later, make him a victim of Alzheimer's disease, particularly if the doctor making the prediction says that he can do nothing to spare him that fate, in the present state of scientific advancement.

(vii) In the West, references are made to *human dignity*. However, one must also speak of the *sacredness* of every human, animal or plant life, as taught by the ancient civilization of India and the cultures that are based upon the unity and uniqueness of nature. "*Man - that useless passion*", Jean-Paul Sartre was wont to say. If that same man knows how to leave life behind him, he will not be that "*useless passion*". What is more, he will hardly be that "*recent invention doomed to an imminent demise*" - the fate kindly predicted for him by Michel Foucoult. Even though ephemeral, he will remain what he always has been - the marvel of creation.

16

CANCER, AIDS, AND QUALITY OF LIFE

Robert N. Butler

International Longevity Center - U.S.
Department of Geriatrics and Adult Development

My thoughts concerning dying and death reflect my experience as a gerontologist, physician and researcher.

As is well known, the industrialized world has gained some 25 years of life expectancy in this century. This twentieth century revolution in longevity is not enjoyed to the same degree in the developing world and yet 60% of all persons over 65 reside there.

Death, then, has become the business of old age. Eighty percent of all deaths occur after age 60 in the developed world. This results from the remarkable reductions in maternal, childhood and infant mortality rates, and, in the past several decades, from drops in death rates after age 65.

In the United States, considerable public anxiety has developed over the character of death. Will physicians adequately relieve pain? Are hospitals too antiseptic? Are the Intensive Care Unit and a variety of technologies overused? Public interest in the subject has been mobilized, in part, by Derek Humphries of the Hemlock Society whose book *Exit* provided information concerning means of committing suicide. Dr. Jack Kevorkian, a retired pathologist in Detroit, Michigan, has promoted physician-assisted suicide. Doubtless there are similar concerns elsewhere in the world. After all, how to die is understandably a major moral and emotional issue, one of the great concerns of our times.

One recent American response has been the founding of the Project on Death in America (PDIA) dedicated to the transformation of the culture and experience of dying. This is supported by the philanthropist and financier, George Soros, through his Open Society Institute. We need to conceptualize quality of dying as well as quality of life. This must be a universal desideratum. At minimum, this means that palliative medicine and nursing must be taught and integrated throughout all contemporary medicine and nursing. But more than that, each of us needs to deal with the personal, existential and spiritual aspects of the end of life and need the support to do so.

If it is true that modern medicine has made death more difficult, need that be so? We have all seen good examples of how medicine can help. Modern medicine, after all, and modern technology as well, bring much relief of pain and other discomforts including, for instance, air hunger, which is so frightening. It was not possible in the past, when natural and unexpected death was so often horrible, to assuage pain, other discomforts, and suffering. Some argue that in modern medicine, doctors view death as a failure; further, that it is impossible to be simultaneously devoted to extending life while assisting those whose life is about to end. But isn't it possible to hold two distinct ideas in the mind at the same time? Sir Francis Bacon, one of the great philosophers of modern science, favored both the scientific efforts to prolong life and, simultaneously, promotion of the "good death" or euthanasia, in its earliest meaning.

At the time of both the American and French Revolutions the average life expectancy was 35. At that time, what we now call Alzheimer's disease and the public called senility was considered a natural part of aging. So, too, many diseases were considered natural, inevitable, unpreventable and untreatable. I would hope we can avoid, on the one hand, the denial of the finitude of life; that is death, and, on the other hand, not give into death prematurely and unnecessarily.

17

ANGUISH AND SUFFERING IN THE FACE OF THE HOSPITAL ORGANIZATIONAL PATTERN

Jean-Michel Lassaunière

Palliative Care Center
Hôtel-Dieu de Paris, Paris

In the fifties, for most of the cancers, the rate of survival was low. As the cancer diagnosis was not disclosed to the patients, the accompaniment of those who were to die was entrusted to groups of religious inspiration. Between the eighties and the nineties, our society has experienced a revolution without precedent in the history of medicine. The first encouraging results were observed in the treatment of cancer and epidemiological studies showed the importance of changes in a number of life factors such as excessive smoking. Psychiatrists and social workers started playing a part in the care to patients, and the hospice movement (1) was initiated in Great Britain and was concerned with the treatment of cancer pain. As early as in 1984, the World Health Organization emphasized the need to treat cancer pain and in 1989, palliative care became integrated as a means in the struggle against cancer (2). It is now possible to define four distinct phases in cancer prevention (3):

1. Disease prevention through education.
2. Advanced disease prevention through early diagnosis programs.
3. Death prevention through disease treatment.
4. Suffering prevention through supportive and palliative care.

The hospital institution must quickly be geared to these changes which is to generate a state of crisis. The anguish and suffering of the patients concerned by cancer treatment and the end of life affect the attending personnel at work. Patients' quality of life requires that the attending personnel take into consideration these psychological and existential dimensions. This fact has an impact on the psychological and physical equilibrium of such a personnel. But it is chiefly the way in which people work together within the institution which can help to manage better the stress related to the treatment of serious diseases.

Cancer, AIDS, and Quality of Life, edited by Levy *et al.*
Plenum Press, New York, 1997

1. HISTORY OF THE STRUGGLE AGAINST CANCER

In 1800, cancer was an incurable and constantly fatal disease. Surgeons started to struggle against cancer thanks to the progress made in anaesthesia (1829: total hysterectomy on a cancer by Récamier, 1890: enlarged mammectomy by Halsted). With the discovery of the ionizing radiation effects on cancer, physics and physicists, non-medical men, entered the hospital. Philanthropists were to be approached for the purchase of a few milligrams of radium. Subsequently, in the fifties, the synthesis of the first alkylating agents inaugurated the era of chemotherapy. In 1992, cancer was recognized as a disorder affecting normal cells and responsible for genetic changes beyond the control of normal regulating systems and likely to develop resistance to cytotoxic drugs. Due to this propensity of malignant cells to modify their genetic system, the cancerous tissue becomes quickly made up of a population of different cells with multiple responses to growth factors and to treatments.

The nursing nun from 1880 will gradually be replaced by nurses trained by physicians, as testifies in 1876, Dr Bourneville, a deputy at the origin of the first free public courses for the staff of the Paris hospitals: *"Our common aim, which we have never deviated from, for twenty five years was to train devoted, educated and skillful nurses, while taking great care to avoid making them believe that they might be able to substitute themselves for the physicians to whom they should remain strictly obedient assistants. Their own interest and the patients' superior interest are at stake"* (4). During the sixties, in the United States, social workers and psychiatrists highlighted the significance of considering jointly the needs of patients, families and attending personnel (5). A new discipline thus was born, namely: psychosocial oncology (6). Since 1967, the Anglo-Saxon palliative care movement originated in Saint Christopher's hospice (1), near London, marked a stage towards the medical support to those who cannot be cured of cancer, while laying emphasis on pluridisciplinarity and pain treatment. More recently, quality of life appears to be a criterion in the comparison of anti-cancer treatments, just as survival.

2. THE INCURABLES

The history of the incurables is explained in detail in P. Pinell's recent book (7). Until the Second World War, the physicians involved in hospital cancerology were not concerned with the lot of the patients suffering from general cancer. As soon as they were incurable, they were regarded as "dregs of society". *"As soon as the disease is considered as incurable, the terms of the exchange are modified, the patient comes under palliative care which **do no longer require any actions from the physician** and which is long-term. Similarly, the patient offers no more interest from a medical point of view. All these factors predispose the clinicians to consider him as a person devoid of any social interest"*(7). The physicians' task focused on localized cancer, which could be cured. Anti-cancer centers were also referred to as "curing plants". Incurables were either sent to "depots" of the Assistance Publique (Health and Social Security services) or left at home in uncomfortable slums with no water and where families were packed, or in Christian charitable organizations (the most important of which had been the "Dames du Calvaire", since 1842). Voluntary lay ladies from the assistance section of the league against cancer tackled the doctors about what they considered as genuine injustice. The incurable cancer sufferer has the right to be given care in order to be relieved of pain.

Since 1930, the notion of incurability has been questioned in favour of a probabilistic vision of the curing chances. After the Second World War and the subsequent Nuremberg trial (8), concerns about the patients' rights appeared in the hospital medicine reforms.

3. THE RELATIONSHIP DIMENSION IN THE CARE

For centuries, hospital medicine had hinged on a tacit agreement implying that in exchange for free care, the poor had to give their body for medical research. Medical knowledge was built up based on this agreement. After the Second World War, the relationship with the patient rested on a paternalistic intention: *"In the presence of the inert and passive patient, the physician has in no way the feeling to be dealing with a free person, an equal, a peer he could actually inform. In his view, any patient is and should be like a child to be tamed"* (9). Nowadays, the relationship is gradually turning towards a behaviour advocating the patient's autonomy (also referred to as the informative pattern). From this relationship, more detailed information emerges about what the patient experiences, for instance in terms of pain or psychological suffering. Based on such information, physicians start showing interest for the psychological aspect of the care and for pain treatment. The consequences of cancer development and death proximity require that the attending personnel (10) be trained both in the psychological dimension of the patient suffering from a serious disease and in improved communication. Psychotherapies whether individual, for patient groups or families are intended to provide, in addition to conventional treatments a better quality of life or of survival. More recently, the legal framework for human experimentation originates the need for the patient's collaboration in a minimum relationship: information given as to the disease, investigations, treatments and enlightened consent. The assertion of the person and of the respect he deserves, as well as of his rights during his stay in a hospital bring about some legal changes (11–15).

4. THE SUFFERING OF THE ATTENDING PERSONNEL

In 1988, French psychoanalyst E. Goldenberg (16), based on his experience with attending teams, mentioned the "suffering of the attending staff" as a new element to be taken into account: *"In the face of death which is always a misfortune, suffering is revealed and expressed. In this context, the nursing staff acquire a genuinely human dimension. They are neither saints, nor demiurges, not even threatening devils, but appear to be instead, in pursuit of the meaning of their work, in search of the causes of the confusion they feel"*. In the Anglo-Saxons countries, as early as in 1975, the stress level of the nurses regularly looking after cancer patients was twice as high as that of their colleagues in other departments. These nurses showed physical and psychological disorders (tiredness, headaches, insomnia, appetite disorders, powerlessness feeling, concentration difficulties) (17–18). These facts have been confirmed more recently in France, by a study about nurses' stress (19). The follow-up and the repeated death of patients constitute the major stress factor but the functioning of the department organized around the physician may constitute an aggravating factor. Another work carried out on the supporting of AIDS sufferers (20) highlights the care organization crisis for those reaching the end of their life: *"There are not yet, in the face of the repeated deaths, team collective behaviours either with physicians or with nurse auxiliaries: it is primarily the nurses who have to bear the hardship of the patients death"*. The compartmentalization between departments and between the professionals of the same department, the lack of communication between professionals, about the working out of care projects for the patients are the main stress factors. Within the context of the training courses we provide, nurses and nurse auxiliaries suffer from the fact that the physicians with whom they are working do not feel concerned with pain evaluation and relief and with specific problems in connection with the approach of their patients' death. They also ask for a participation into the decisions regarding the patients at the end of their life. In the absence of such a discussion, it seems to them that they are executing prescriptions comparable to prolongation of life with medical means. Such demands reflect a need for recognition of their role and a need for autonomy with respect to the medical profession. (*"The nurse behaved like a good housewife subjected to her husband... Anyway, it is no more a question now of relations between a physician and HIS nurse"*. (21). In her recent book, M. Ruzsniewski (22) based on her experience as a psychologist in a hematology department and in the palliative care center of the Hôtel-Dieu, shows how the nurses' and the patients' defense mechanisms operate in order to limit the anguish impact. She says that nurses *"are therefore bound to admit that the group alone, owing to its intrinsic dynamics and its entity, can make it possible to alleviate the confusion and the anguish due to such a crucial questioning, unceasingly repeated at each stage of the disease: what could possibly be done when recovery becomes an illusion?"*. The group link within the institution has to be found again and a **nurse community** has to be created in order to bear better the weight of the anguish related to the uncertainty between living and dying, that patients, families and nurses feel.

The suffering of the attending staff results also from a greater "proximity" with the patient and his family. The word proximity is to be understood with different meanings. First of all social proximity. Until the end of the Second World War, the access to the hospital was reserved for the indigent, the poorest, the lower classes. Owing to the status of the doctor, who was often regarded as a magician, and to the social gap between him and the patient, the doctor was inevitably kept at arm's length. Similarly, the nun was in the first place in the service of God through her relationship with the patient. Nowadays, the patients and the nursing staff have relations in which class differences are diminished by the development of social classes within society. The profession of physician or nurse in the hospital does no longer arouse much envy from a financial point of view. Nurses can feel a likeness between themselves and the patients they look after and conversely. The representation of suffering has radically changed. In the early twentieth century, suffering was socially perceived as directly connected with hard living conditions. Living, surviving, earning one's living was a fight, a struggle and death a fatality: *"Getting used to the idea of suffering always. An age, a combination of circumstances will come and make of life a perpetual pain. If you did not get accustomed beforehand with the idea that such a situation is awaiting you, you might not have the right frame of mind to undergo it with profit"* - (23).

Nowadays, extended lifetime and improved living conditions resulting from public health and higher standard of living, and the effects on social welfare, are such that suffering has become an unacceptable and outrageous eventuality. Patients are informed about disease prevention, diagnostics and treatment. However such information generates the anguish of suffering and the anguish of death. The announcement of a serious disease diagnosis has psychological consequences and any information of this kind should be accompanied by a support over time so that the psychological adaptation can occur. Proximity should also be understood in the physical meaning of the word. Death frightens. To a physician, a patient who dies means a failure, powerlessness and there is a strong likelihood that the one who is dying be kept at a distance because he is disquieting. Exclusion, rejection by the physician as well as by society which while dismissing death from collective consciousness, rejects the patient who is dying. It is the refusal to exclude them which led nurses to get involved in the accompaniment of the patients where they experience this physical proximity through nursing and touching. The disease and the treatments affect the body and the bodily care allow the patient to take possession again of his body, a suffering body. Proximity is also to be understood in the ethical meaning of the word, in the relationship with others, between the nurse and the nursed. The anguish of the suffering patient is also an appeal for the other's solicitude, in this case for the nurse's solicitude. The nurse community wants to be also a moral community in its responsibility towards the other powerless, suffering and who is going to die (24).

5. DEVELOPMENT OF THE HOSPITAL ORGANIZATION (25)

The hospital encounters some difficulties of adaptation. On the one hand there is the scientific and medical logic, caring more than ever before, about its values of efficiency and rationality, and the administrative logic, which in the context of budget restrictions, lays emphasis on considerations of output, rationalization of tasks and expenses. On the other hand, other values emerge, such as the importance of reception, quality of life, singularity of care. Both these approaches give rise to a twofold requirement, i.e.: nurses have to work profitably, efficiently, they should get involved into corporate dynamics, accept the resulting requirements (staff cuts, increased production and workload, efficient management, quantitative assessment) but they should also personalize care, take time to receive, listen, educate, support and be with the patients and their families through to the end. Within an institution adapting itself slowly, due to the stakes and powers, this results in professional frustration. The constraints are obvious when it comes to the hospital-company approach. If both these terms may appear not to be antinomical, then a new sense has to be defined. If the company pattern may be applied to the hospital one, we still have to achieve more than merely making a transposition in which the finished product would be the treated patient. In other words, we should think about changes to be done in order to meet new specific requirements in the hospital mission. Can the adaptation be achieved through the preparation of a community work, according to the interdisciplinary mode ?

A team is a group of people anxious of working towards a common objective. Each one has a professional skill. The pooling of these multiple skills within the team gives rise to discussions, exchanges, research as well as possible conflicts. These exchanges gradually make each one's skills grow richer. The team's product is greater than the sum of each member's products. The essential condition, so that the team can work properly, lies in the clear definition of the group's rules (structuring) and in the respect of such rules. We health professionals are in most cases handicapped in terms of interdisciplinarity and we reproduce more or less consciously the patterns inherited from the French medical education. We shall probably need one or two generations to see mentalities move towards a more genuine pluridisciplinarity based on the respect for the professionals and their skills. However, such an evolution meets with considerable resistance, and is sometimes perceived as actual subversion by those who are obsessed with the idea of exercising power on the others. The development of palliative care and care structures is a field where interdisciplinarity around the patient is perceptible and as such it arouses significant resistance within the health sector, as a place of subversion.

6. CONCLUSION

The quality of in-patients' end of life calls for a better quality of life for health professionals. The hospital institution has some difficulties in adapting itself to the developing and rapidly-changing needs in terms of health, but it is primarily the relations between professionals which have to be changed so that the patient can actually be at the center of the care. Such a change affects the mentalities of the various actors in the hospital, including the physicians Thereby, anguish will be recognized and expressed in the interest of the nurses, the patients and their families.

REFERENCES

1. Saunders C. The management of terminal malignant disease. Second edition. Edward Arnold (Publishers) Ltd, 1984.
2. Traitement de la douleur et soins palliatifs (Pain treatment and palliative care). Report No. 804 of a committee of experts of the World Health Organization - Geneva 1990.
3. McDonald N. The interface between oncology and palliative medicine *in Oxford Textbook of palliative medicine.* Edited by Doyle D, Hanks GWC and McDonald N. *Oxford Medical Publications.* 1994.
4. Schaeffe D. La profession infirmière (the nurse profession). *Etudes,* March 1989, 370/3: 313–22.
5. Hinton J. Mental and physical distress in the dying. *Quarterly Journal of Medicine.* 1963, 32;1.
6. Holland J.C. Rowland JH. Handbook of Psychooncology. Oxford University Press, New York, 1989.
7. Pinell P. "Naissance d'un fléau, histoire de la lutte contre le cancer en France (1890–1940)" (Birth of a scourge, history of the struggle against cancer in France), Métailié Publications, 1992.
8. Ambroselli C. L'éthique médicale (Medical ethics). Que sais-je. No. 2422. PUF.
9. Portes L. First president of the National Medical Association, paper intended for the Academy of Moral and Political Sciences, 1950.
10. Delvaux N, Razavi D, Farvacques C. Cancer care - a stress for health professionals. *Social and Science Medicine* 27(2), 159–166, 1988.
11. Law No. 88–1138 of December 20, 1988 regarding the protection of persons involved in biomedical research, referred to as Huriet law, amended by law No. 94–630 of July 25, 1994.
12. Law No. 94–653 of July 29 relating to the respect of the human body (French Official Gazette - July 30, 1994).
13. Law No. 94–548 of July 1, 1994, about the processing of name-linked data intended for research in the health field and amending law No. 78–17 of January 6, 1978 about data processing, files and freedom (French official gazette of July 2, 1994).
14. Law No. 95–116 of February 4, 1995 regarding a number of social measures as to pain treatment.
15. Statement about the promotion of patients' rights in Europe. Amsterdam, March 28–30, 1994.
16. Goldenberg E. Aider les soignants en souffrance (Help suffering nurses). *JALMALV*; 1988, 14: 3–13.
17. Vachon MLS. Occupational stress in the care of the critically ill, the dying an the bereaved. Washington, Hemisphere Publishing Corporation, 1987.
18. Kash KM, Breitbart W. The stress of caring for cancer patients. In: Psychiatric Aspects of Symptom Management in Cancer Patients (Edited by Breitbart W and Holland JC) p 243–260. American Psychiatric Press, Washington, 1993.
19. Rodary C. Les infirmières. Diagnostic d'épuisement professionnel. (Nurses. Diagnosis of occupational exhaustion). *Etudes,* March 1994, 3803: 323–32.
20. Lert F, Marne MJ. Les soignants et la prise en charge des personnes atteintes de SIDA à l'hôpital (Nurses and caring for AIDS sufferers in the hospital). March 1991. GESTE Laboratory, Public Health, INSERM U88.
21. Michelangeli C, et al. L'infirmière, de la gratitude à la reconnaissance (The nurse, from gratitude to recognition). *Etudes,* March 1993; 383: 317–26.
22. Ruszniewski M. Face à la maladie grave: patients, familles, soignants (In the face of a serious disease: patients, families, nurses). Dunod, Privat. Paris 1995.
23. Une aide dans la douleur, par l'auteur des avis spirituels (A help in pain, by the author of the spiritual advice). Fifth edition. Jules Gervais, Editor 1886.
24. Ricoeur P. Soi-même comme un autre (Oneself like another). 1990. Editions du Seuil, Paris.
25. Lassaunière JM, Plagès B. Les modèles organisationnels à l'hôpital, l'interdisciplinarité (Organizational patterns in the hospital, interdisciplinarity) *JALMALV,* 1995 ; 40: 35–39.

18

LIVING WELL IN THE SHADOW OF DEATH

Joanne Lynn

Center to Improve Care of the Dying
The George Washington University
1001 22nd St. NW, Suite 820
Washington, DC 20037

Only two generations ago, most people, in what are now economically advantaged countries, still died young and quickly. They lived no more than a few hours or days with knowledge of their impending death. Even with cancer, people died (at any age) in just a short time, with tasks incomplete, and with at best the opportunity to say farewells and make peace with God. Now, except for trauma and AIDS, most of us in developed countries will die in old age of an illness that will progressively disable and afflict us over years.

This new reality follows an era in which, at least in the United States, we avoided noticing the facts of irreversibly progressive illness and death. We have mislaid whatever stories might once have made sense of dying. We do talk of death, but only in the very elderly or those very obviously near dying. In fact, that observation is relevant to cancer and AIDS. Among ways to die, these are unusual though paradigmatic. They have a discernible terminal phase and the time to death is usually fairly predictable. As Klastersky's presentation illustrates, we do not even know for sure what we would want to measure in assessing how well we care for people at the end of life.

By all accounts, we are not doing very well no matter how one measures it. Laussauniere's presentation outlines some of the shortcomings. Our recent Study to Understand Prognoses and Preferences for Outcomes and Risks of Treatments (SUPPORT)[1] describes the dying of over 4000 seriously ill patients. Half of the families, interviewed after the deaths of patients who were conscious, reported that the patient had endured severe or moderately severe pain most or all of the time in the days just before death. This level of pain afflicted every disease, not just cancer. Half of our patients who died had spent their last week or more in an intensive care unit. One-third of the families lost most or all of their savings.[2] Three-fourths of these very seriously ill patients did not have any discussion of resuscitation with their physicians. Even among dying patients who said that they would not want resuscitation tried, only about half had any discussion with a hospital physician about the issue. Only about one-tenth had resuscitation tried, but the order to forgo it was usually written in the last three days.

Cancer, AIDS, and Quality of Life, edited by Levy *et al.*
Plenum Press, New York, 1997

The picture is quite disheartening, and much has been said and written about how to improve it. Our first efforts have largely been ineffective. Many think that having patients write a statement about what care they want will make a difference. In the US, this has taken the form of "living wills" which are usually preprinted forms that have some language contending that the patient wants no "heroic" or "artificial" treatments to sustain life when it is clear that death is "imminent" and that treatment can "only prolong dying." Our study found these documents to be singularly ineffective in their present use. They are often not brought to the hospital, less than half are ever discussed with a doctor, and almost none have any more specific instructions, thereby leaving it to someone to interpret the meaning.

Some also think that we could set some statistical threshold of likely survival and try to stop all life-sustaining treatment for those who are so seriously ill. Such a "futility" policy in the SUPPORT population would be difficult to achieve and of modest impact.[3] A threshold of 1% chance of surviving two months, for example, would find 115 patients in 4306, but almost all of these patients die in the next day or two in current care. Only twelve patients accounted for three-quarters of the days of living beyond the day of prognostication, and they were young, with good prior function, and wanting treatment. They would be the hardest cases in which to allow a statistical threshold to have an effect. Yet, without applying it to them, there is no real effect at all.

We thought that major inroads might be gained by making it easy to discuss the issues early in hospitalization. We set out to provide excellent information about prognosis and about the patient and family understanding and preferences. We provided a skilled nurse to help carry on and precipitate the discussions. The intervention was successfully implemented. The SUPPORT intervention had no substantial impact upon the patients' experience or on the decision-making.

This was an eye-opening finding. Courts, commentators, leading physicians, codes of ethics, and guidelines for practice in the U.S. had goaded health care to do exactly what we did. Was there no interest in change? Were physicians just blind to the problems? What had gone wrong?

Definitive answers to that question await further work, but there are some interesting observations that might lead the way.

First, patients and families were eager for information and counseling, but did not have strong views on how they should be treated. Indeed, patients and families were similarly satisfied whether they got what they claimed to want or not. Many patients affirmatively turned down the opportunity to say that they wanted to talk with their physician about the use of resuscitation.

Secondly, physicians and everyone involved had strong patterns of care that seemed adequate. Each physician thought that his or her practice was probably acceptable, even though the average practices were troubling. There was little motivation for change.

Thirdly, there were much stronger forces sustaining routine practices than we expected. For example, we were intrigued to find that our five hospitals varied widely in how often persons were at home to die, and how often in the hospital.[4] The adjusted odds ratio spanned nearly five times the likelihood of dying at home for one hospital as compared with another. This was almost not correlated with sociodemographic, physiologic, or preference descriptors of the populations at each hospital. However, when we looked at the rates of dying at home among our nation's elderly Medicare population, a very interesting correlation arose. Measures of the use and availability of hospital beds in the geographic region have a profound correlation with the rates at which people die at home or in hospitals. About two-third of the variation in site of death is explained by hospitalization rates for Medicare beneficiaries. Most likely, in areas with high rates of in-hospital death, we are seeing not just the effects of building hospitals and having developed the habit of using them, but also the effects of not having adequate supply of well-integrated home care and hospice care. The effect is so strong that one could hardly have hoped that any one patient and physician could have made changes in a system that is "used to" keeping patients in the hospital, or that is "used to" sending them home.

Fourthly, we are seeing a substantial effect of age on aggressiveness of care in the population over 65 years old. First noted by Lubitz et al,[5] we are prone to spend much more on the last year of persons who die in their 60's and 70's than on persons who die in their 80's and beyond. In SUPPORT, we have seen that age affects the likelihood of having an order against trying resuscitation, with it being more than three times as likely to have an order at 85 than at 55, even after adjustment for prognosis and preferences.[6] Likewise, even after adjustment for clinical condition and indications for treatments, we are seeing a substantial diminution in the rates of specific interventions with age, including hospitalization itself, dialysis, and surgery .[7, 8] This is an interesting cultural pattern, as it indicates that we do know "how to stop" in more elderly patients. Perhaps the definition of a reasonable life span, and their having exceeded that expectation, is a strong shaper of the behaviors of caregivers and families, influencing the course of care in largely inarticulate ways.

Finally, we have found that the designation of a patient as "dying" occurs fairly late in the course of disease. It seems that the physicians and the culture generally have some understanding of when that is appropriate, and that the designation occurs fairly late in the course of persons with illnesses studied by SUPPORT. The public believes that we know how to prognosticate death, and probably even physicians believe that they know who will die soon. A new analysis we are doing belies that claim. For 100 patients who will actually die on Saturday, the median prognosis on Friday is about one in ten to survive two months. On Thursday, the median prognosis is up to about one in four, and on Wednesday it is up to one in three. This means that the usual patient who dies on Saturday still seems to have a real chance to survive a substantial time on Wednesday. We are not in the habit of talking about death until the odds are really stacked against us, and one in three or four may not seem bad enough. Thus, discussions are delayed for a day or two, and this obviates the opportunity to make decisions to focus upon spiritual matters, or pain control, or on being at home.

The situation in the United States is changing rapidly, and mostly for the better. Various private foundations are supporting work to improve care. The public is beginning to demand more information and better care. The prestigious Institute of Medicine has launched a study. The American Medical Association has announced a priority for research, education, and improved reimbursement for this work, along with an official recognition of how little has been done.[9] The Project on Death in America, a branch of the Open Society Institute, has funded two dozen leaders in medicine and a few dozen research or demonstration projects, aiming to catalyze reform. The Robert Wood Johnson Foundation is leading a major effort to improve public education and mobilize affected organizations. The background changes toward severe constraints in medical care funding and capitated modes of payment have created new vulnerabilities for the seriously ill and dying. Time will tell whether we can learn to provide the care system that grants meaning to the end of life, or whether we will learn to accept a much more grim end of life.

In the polite language of the day, there are many opportunities for improvement. We are not doing well and even minimal attention to the subject is likely to lead to improvements. As we deal with quality of life at its end, we must learn to handle the fact that the end is not fixed in time. Clearly, one way to change quality of life would be to have euthanasia widespread. This issue will undoubtedly divide thoughtful people and frequently divert us from more important issues.

The power of achieving change through mobilizing patients seems likely to be modest. It seems much more likely that we can achieve change through restructuring the care system, its cues to patients, and the expectations of providers. In the long run, it is inadequate to improve care of cancer and AIDS patients near death without improving long term care and the care of the dying generally. Although we in the U.S. have managed to create a rather privileged care system for cancer and AIDS in hospice, that is likely to be a prime target as the care system becomes much less wealthy.

Of course, we may still be asking the wrong questions and seeking the wrong reforms. Perhaps what matters to dying persons is more often their social role and relationships and their meaningfulness. We may not achieve important reform until we can find ways to cherish the disabled and ill, and to love those near death. And these are conditions that are not easily prescribed.

REFERENCES

1. The SUPPORT Principal Investigators. A controlled trial to improve care for seriously ill hospitalized patients: The Study to Understand Prognoses and Preferences for Outcomes and Risks of Treatments (SUPPORT). JAMA 1995;274:1591-1598.
2. Covinsky KE, Goldman L, Cook EF, Oye R, Reding D, Fulkerson W, Connors AF, Lynn J, Phillips RS: The impact of serious illness on patients' families. JAMA 1994;272,:1939-1844.
3. Teno JM, Murphy D, Lynn J, Tosteson A, Desbiens N, Connors A, Hamel MB, Wu A, Phillips R, Wenger N, Harrell F,Jr., Knaus WA, for the SUPPORT Investigators: Prognosis-based futility guidelines: Does anyone win? J Am Geriatr Soc 1994;42:1202-1207.
4. Pritchard R, Teno J, Fisher E, Lynn J, Phillips RS, Reding D, Fulkerson W, Wenger N, for the SUPPORT Investigators. Regional variation in the place of death. J Gen Intern Med 9:146a, 1994.
5. Lubitz J, Beebe J, Backer C. Longevity and medicare expenditures. New England Journal of Medicine. 1995;332:999-1003
6. Lynn J, Teno J, Wenger N, Phillips R, Wu A, Connors A, Youngner S, Layde P. "Do not resuscitate orders" in seriously ill patients: Expressed preferences or last rites? Clin Res 1992;40(2):347a.
7. Layde PM, Beam CA, Bruste SK, Connors AF, Desbiens N, Lynn J, Phillips RS, Reding D, Teno J, Vidallet H, Wenger N. Surrogates' predictions of seriously ill patients' resuscitation preferences (in press), Archives of Family Mediciene.
8. Hamel, MB, Golman L, Teno JM, Lynn J, Connors AF, Galanos A, Desbiens N, Reding D, Oye RK, Phillips RL for the SUPPORT Investigators. Patient age and hospital resource use. J Gen Intern Med. 1994;9(suppl):43. Abstract.
9. Council on Scientific Affairs, AMA. Council report: Good care of the dying patient. JAMA 1996; 275.

19

QUALITY OF LIFE

Cultural, Socio-Economic, and Geographic Perspectives

Eka Esu-Williams

Society of Women and AIDS in Africa (SWAA)
Family Health International
AIDS Control and Prevention Project
1601 Adeola Hopewell St.
Victoria Island
Lagos, Nigeria

INTRODUCTION

In discussing the socio-economic and cultural dimensions of quality of life, a global analysis will be inappropriate because of the complexities and differences in culture and economies between geographic areas. This paper will focus on experiences from Nigeria within an African context which could be applicable to other regions of the developing world with similar socio-economic and cultural settings. This approach is likely to bring issues into focus more clearly than using the developed, western world as the basis for discussing socio-economic and cultural factors of quality of life. Overall, the paper is intended to provide a basis for a broad-based discussion and interest from diverse groups such as medical professionals who often do not accommodate social and cultural dimensions of quality of life and others who are unaware of, poorly informed about or not involved in enunciating quality of life issues. Whereas quality of life concepts have been recognized and medical practice to incorporate them promoted in developed countries, in developing countries, the main priority centers around the provision of treatment and care for patients, in anticipation of possible cure.

Using cancer and HIV/AIDS to examine quality of life highlights the extent to which socio-economic and cultural factors and physical-biological factors are interdependent. They also illustrate the complexity of socio-cultural factors, and the diverse ways they may influence perceptions of and responses to different terminal conditions. Because of the magnitude of the HIV/AIDS epidemic in Africa, its many facets and implications have become evident. In comparison with cancer, HIV/AIDS is more stigmatized and portends greater negative socio-cultural and economic implications. HIV/AIDS therefore enables us to identify a wider range of quality of life issues and to consider responses

Cancer, AIDS, and Quality of Life, edited by Levy *et al.*
Plenum Press, New York, 1997

towards improving the lives of terminally ill patients. Though broader, many of the issues raised by HIV/AIDS in respect of quality of life are applicable to cancer. This paper will therefore concentrate primarily on some of the lessons gained from HIV/AIDS within an African socio-economic and cultural context.

TOWARDS A DEFINITION OF QUALITY OF LIFE

It may prove to be too complex to try to define and measure quality of life between individuals and groups across cultures and geographic areas. It is also difficult to formulate concepts and identify determinants that can be measured appropriately in populations from different countries and cultures and even within the same country where there are wide socio-economic differences. Since social and cultural norms and values are important in every society and many countries are implementing economic policies which cannot guarantee adequate care/support for chronically ill patients, we need to ascertain what we mean and understand by quality of life and what is possible to offer and to access by those affected. It has been recognized that there are universal phenomena which relate to health and disease but which are not culture-bound. The nature of these is likely to be the biological and physiological characteristics of human beings. But in considering the more personal and abstract aspects of life, socio-economic and cultural factors become relevant as the key determinants in establishing priorities for patients.

To meet biological, social and cultural needs of patients, defining quality of life requires that we place a great emphasis on what patients, families and communities perceive to be important rather than that prescribed by health professionals. A definition of quality of life incorporating social and cultural values and concerns will make it imperative to diagnose and manage chronic life-threatening diseases not only from a medical stance, but will demand that we predict and respond to non-medical outcomes capable of impacting well-being.

Quality of life should not be separated from the life which one lives in relation to family and community and the attendant health services and infrastructure, influenced or partially determined by the socio-economic state of the individual and community. Also, the individual may have a personal conviction about what state of well-being is measured by and how his/her own life may be considered accomplished. For instance, for many persons marriage and procreation constitute a key priority and living then becomes important in order to support one's children and family. Perception of quality of life during terminal illness is often linked to one's ability to accomplish his/her life's priorities and responsibilities, and to secure the guarantee for important personal/family matters to be taken care of when death occurs.

MEDICAL VERSUS SOCIO-ECONOMIC AND CULTURAL PERSPECTIVES OF QUALITY OF LIFE

The concept, content and assessment of quality of life within a health context have focused overwhelmingly on the ability of a person to accomplish physical activities, to continue with occupational and social roles and to a lesser extent conform with some culturally relevant attributes of well-being. Therefore, the health model of quality of care is focused on the individual and on matters perceived to be a priority to the individual. This individualistic medical viewpoint assumes that physical, social and mental functional capacity of a person can be equated to well-being. A socio-cultural viewpoint de-emphasizes on the individual. Rather, it looks at the many components of the individual's environment and his/her ability to be a functional part of that environment.

Our current knowledge of quality of life is still very much a western medical concept which is alien to even medical professionals in developing countries. And because we are largely confined to medically defined and researched paradigms, I believe that one of the most critical questions to address in seeking to examine a broader perspective of quality of life is, whether we can reach agreement about a common global notion that is acceptable and understandable within different environments. If we can evolve a universally accepted and understood notion, one major concern also would be how factors derived from different socio-economic and cultural environments would affect the ability to achieve a common goal. This is bound to be a tremendous challenge. Already the HIV/AIDS epidemic has provided insight on the extent to which socio-economic and cultural factors can influence the way individuals, communities and even governments perceive and respond to chronic life-threatening diseases. The epidemic has further increased our appreciation of how socio-economic and cultural factors can be disenabling or supportive in the quest to improve quality of life.

Understanding and responding to quality of life issues from a socio-economic and cultural context mean that we need to take into account profound differences between people in perceptions, expectations, values, and priorities regarding life and death, and furthermore, how these differences may affect decision-making during terminal illness. Quality of life thus needs to be looked at in connection with a specific disease - how the disease is perceived and how care-support can be provided. For instance what is the implication for quality of life if a patient speaks openly about his HIV/AIDS condition within a cultural atmosphere where the disease is highly stigmatized and a socio-economic environment where access to care and treatment is very limited?

We can look at the impact of society and culture on life threatening diseases and thus quality of life in two ways. Firstly, prevalent social attitudes and cultural beliefs influence the way in which certain disease conditions are perceived. Regarding HIV/AIDS, social stigma attached to the condition has contributed in many ways to undermine care-support efforts for those affected. Secondly, it has been demonstrated that chronic terminal disease (especially where experienced at an epidemic level), can impact on socio-economic and cultural aspects of life- impeding societal and cultural developments, engendering economic hardships at many levels and exacerbating the disease situation as well. These two mutually related impacts affect quality of life. Interestingly, these socially and culturally influenced perceptions and responses have not remained static. Where appropriate interventions have been applied, negative tendencies have been modified or changed in such a manner that they have enhanced quality of life of patients. For example, through the determined efforts of health providers and activists, individual and groups of people living with HIV/AIDS, societal stigma has reduced, and the care of patients at home and in community has become widespread and more acceptable to many communities in Africa and elsewhere.

Though a shift in concept of quality of life, has occurred in many parts of the world over the last two years from the healthy to the sick and vulnerable, in a social and economically depressed environment, this transition is unrealistic. The quality of life of the "well" which is still subject to rapid deterioration is a matter of grave concern. How does the poor state of the "well" affect the decision made regarding those with terminal illness? The concept of quality of life it appears needs to stem from a backdrop of socio-economic and cultural conditions, in which what happens to people in "good health" affects the way in which people respond to quality of life concerns terminally ill patients.

SOCIAL, CULTURAL, AND ECONOMIC FACTORS, AND QUALITY OF LIFE

Given the intensity of its HIV/AIDS epidemic, Africa probably provides one of the most valid opportunities to examine extensively the interaction between quality of life, terminal illnesses and socio-economic and cultural factors. Socio-economic conditions have determined to a large extent how medical professionals, individuals, families and communities perceive and respond to HIV/AIDS. Social, economic and cultural factors can play positive or negative roles in determining quality of life for terminally ill patients. Class and gender can compound the negative impact of these factors. However, a window of opportunity also exists to change these factors where they are negative towards increasing the level of care and support for patients.

In many parts of Africa the poor economic climate, an acute epidemic of HIV/AIDS has weakened the already ailing health systems and health providers, weary of the risk of infection are reluctant to provide care. There are limited viable options for palliative care and reliance on conventional medical treatment is often of necessity de-emphasized because it is usually inaccessible, unaffordable or non-existent. Its quality is not comparable with what obtains in many developed countries due to poor health infrastructure and inadequate resources. It is difficult to determine how quality of life for the terminally ill can be enhanced under such health systems. Therefore, treatment for life-threatening, chronic health problems is anchored on traditional remedies and home care. This points to the fact that medicine and medical care are much more broadly-defined in Africa than in the developed world. They incorporate the services of western-trained medical practitioners, traditional herbalists, local healers, religious leaders and family members. Strategies to improve quality of life of patients should focus on these various sources of patient care.

Gender and social status often influence the commitment of families and communities to provide care and support during illness. In general, illness in women tends to receive less priority and attention compared to that of men. The man is accorded greater priority because he is seen as the family head, the breadwinner and believed to be fundamental to family continuity. Ironically, women are the major providers of care to the terminally ill, but lack access to health care and, if ill themselves can hardly expect to be properly looked after by family members. They and their family members often do not accord priority to their health needs and problems. Because of women's numerous responsibilities, lack of support and resources they tend to neglect their health problems. Thus, from a gender perspective, women suffer a dual effect in relation to care. Culturally, the question of quality of life has a gender dimension. This is based on how the lives of men and women are differently perceived and valued. Added to these gender-linked perceptions, cultural expectations in many parts of Africa place a great emphasis on procreation and the need to be survived by offsprings. This pressurizes HIV infected women to have children, thus compromising their health status. Women are in a bind regarding the enhancement of their well-being during terminal illness.

Superstition and stigma associated with HIV/AIDS (but far less with cancers) have curtailed options for appropriate response. Stigma is often directed more intensely on women. Both stigma and superstition influence greatly the manner in which diseases are perceived and responded to. Even to be said of health workers is the fact they are primarily the product of specific cultural and societal systems and in dealing with patients with stigmatized illness, they tend to exhibit prevailing attitudinal tendencies, especially where they have not been properly sensitized. This is even more so when medical professionals have limited skills and materials to manage patients with contagious infections. For example, patients with incurable, life threatening diseases in Nigeria are often told by doctors and nurses that "their disease is not a matter for hospital treatment". This tends to shift attention from hospital care to other channels of care, some of which may not necessarily be beneficial to the patient.

Culturally, death of the aged is considered to be natural and regarded as a call to join the ancestors. It is generally not mourned and could be celebrated depending on the social and traditional status of the dead. A link between the living and dead is acknowledged in many cultures and traditionally families and communities treat the dying with dignity because it is believed that their spirits provide protection for the living. In contrast, illness and death of the young (as is experienced with AIDS) is considered unnatural and evoke a lot of superstition and crisis. Premature death is judged to be an ill-omen, a result of a curse or other causes. Quite often enormous and scarce resources are committed in seeking to find the "source/origin" of illness rather than providing care and support for the patient, while also neglecting the well-being of other family members.

Traditionally, care for the sick is rooted in family and community structures with the immediate and extended families playing a significant role. Improving the quality of life is compatible with the African value system which ensures that the pain of illness and death is shared by relatives and friends. The family-community approach for care emphasizes love, affection and emotional, spiritual and material support. The HIV/AIDS epidemic provides the opportunity to advocate for the rights of patients to quality care, and for their quality of life to be enhanced through social and economic empowerment of families and communities. This is important in order to increase acceptance and care for the terminally ill no matter the type of disease encountered. This family-community based care system is threatened, unfortunately, by adverse socio-economic factors and modernization which is eroding cultural belief systems, while promoting alien values and lifestyles. For example, tradition demands that the sick and dying are cared for and treated with dignity. Many people are now unable to fulfil this obligation because they are poor themselves or because traditional values no longer appeal to them or they have lost touch with their our traditions.

In many countries particularly in Africa, health infrastructure, level of motivation of health providers, available resources and facilities constitute a major obstacle in providing adequate care and support for terminally ill patients. Hospitals are often the last resort of patients and families because the cost of treatment is unaffordable and the chances of recovery not considered encouraging. Prolonged states of adverse economic factors, especially widespread poverty have worsened the quality of life of most people in developing countries. The situation is aggravated by lopsided allocation of scare resources - resulting in grossly inadequate social and health services. Key services required to improve health care and quality life for citizens are non existent or of poor quality. The ability to access health care is linked with the ability to procure services and treatment. Implementing a medically-oriented and evaluated quality of life determinants under these conditions constitutes a major challenge for health professional.

CONCLUSION

The current medically conceptualized framework of quality of life provides a theoretical basis for global understanding and action, but to be more relevant, its contents and practice need to be linked with socio-cultural and economic specificities. The medical concept also should be regarded as an important tool for up-grading the quality of care patients receive during terminal illness and for improving overall commitment to the care of the sick. This goal is paramount for developing countries where patient care is yet to be a priority of governments.

The prevailing state of our health care systems and structures can offer only limited viable options for palliative and curative care for the terminally ill. The family-community framework and non-governmental organizations provide the most sustainable channels for promoting the quality of care and life of the terminally ill, but they must be strengthened and mobilized in order to cope with the magnitude of the problem and for sustaining long-term action. The debate around the quality of life at the community level must address such critical issues as the rights and participation of patients in decisions about their lives. It must also articulate the role and responsibilities of health providers in promoting quality of care and life of the terminally ill and also how to deal with the problem of stigma and superstition.

Given that generally quality of life tends to be viewed as being culture neutral, its cultural and socio-economic dimensions need to be vigorously explored and appreciated. This approach will as of necessity encompass the medical, family and community contributions to quality of life of patients within their socio-economic and cultural environment.

Socio-cultural perspectives of quality of life provide us the opportunity to redefine priorities for patient care and support during terminal illness. Eliciting and respecting the wishes of the patient are no less important factors in promoting his/her emotional and physical well-being and dignity. This approach will also allow us to address practices which adversely affect dependents of patients such as property inheritance by widows and children. The inability of women and children to have access to property has constituted a major crisis in many communities ravaged by HIV/AIDS in Africa, reducing the quality of life of survivors.

To promote effectively the principles and practice of quality of life, we need to focus attention on dealing more effectively with stigma and superstition. Verbal engagement by patients with HIV/AIDS is a new dimension in health care, giving opportunity for orientation of health politics, research, and prevention. A lot of difficulties are still experienced in utilizing this approach in Africa because of cultural sensitivities. Stigma apart, bad news such as of terminal illness is guarded with secrecy because of the potential negative social implications such as unsuitability for marriage, erroneous belief that the patient carries an undesirable genetic disease and the possibility of worsening condition if disease is perceived to be caused by human or spiritual agents.

To conclude, the medical objectives and principles of quality of life are important and desirable within a social and cultural context where well-being can be improved. It cannot be used effectively for promoting a rigorous, research-oriented medical approach to quality of care. It can form a basis for promoting inputs and collaboration among patients, family, medical and related experts. It is obvious that the current social and economic development system, particularly the health care system is handicapped and cannot sustain the quality of care that is desirable for the terminally ill in many countries. Thus quality of life of the terminally ill must be defined within the support systems of the family and community, while identifying and improving upon what hospitals and medical professionals can effectively provide.

20

QUALITY OF LIFE

Socio-Economic, Geographic, and Cultural Factors

Lieve Fransen

Commission of the European Communities
AIDS Task Force
Rue de Genève 10, Box 7
B-1140 Brussels, Belgium

This paper presents some discussion points examining quality of life in its socio-economic context and highlights some of the enormous imbalances in choices and opportunities between different parts of the world. Some people do not have drinking water, or adequate food or shelter: is this related to our questions about quality of life?

The discussion is divided in three parts:

- 1. *First* a demonstration that the relation between quality of life, health and socio-economic position is positive and progressive and that health inequalities are universal between countries and in countries: the relation between health and wealth.
- 2. *Secondly*, an examination of some of the directions taken by:
- 2.1. the ongoing, worldwide, social reforms and
- 2.2. the lessons from the HIV epidemic.
- 3. *In the third part* some conclusions are brought forward.

Before developing these three areas, it is useful to give an idea on how the terminology regarding quality of life, and poverty is used in this paper:

- Quality of life is determined and achieved through a balance between the presence of elements such as health, knowledge, education, income, positive environments and social infrastructure. This is true at individual and at societal levels.
- Poverty or the opposite of wealth could be defined, not just as the lack of income, but the lack of quality of life related to the lack of such resources as income, health, knowledge, education, and positive environments. This puts greater emphasis on human capital beyond the sole focus on economic capital.

The articulation of these definitions is important in order to set the stage for the discussion. 'Quality of life' is an *equilibrium* between different elements (Figure 1). It is in this context that we can understand how individuals and communities make trade-offs be-

Cancer, AIDS, and Quality of Life, edited by Levy *et al.*
Plenum Press, New York, 1997

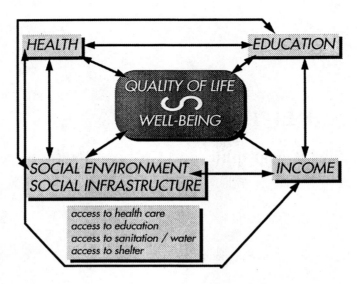

Figure 1. Elements determining quality of life.

tween the elements that produce well-being. Rather than pursue maximum health or education, people make choices pursuing optimal health to achieve well-being and this is true in different socio-economic contexts.

1. HOW THE RELATIONSHIP BETWEEN QUALITY OF LIFE, HEALTH, AND SOCIO-ECONOMIC POSITION IS POSITIVE AND PROGRESSIVE

When examining figures such as those in the World Development Report of the World Bank and the Human Development Report of the United Nations Development Programme (UNDP) (1 & 2), some facts come forward: wealth of a country and of individuals is important and in very broad terms a direct relation is found between wealth, health and health expenditures (Figs. 2–4). When health is measured through indicators such as infant mortality or life expectancy and wealth through an indicator such as the Global Domestic Product (GDP), for example, a direct relationship is found (Fig. 2). Wealth and health themselves are two of the elements facilitating quality of life.

Country	% of GDP	Health outcome	Infant mortality
Japan	6.5 %	best	5/1000
France	9 %	middle	7/1000
USA	12 %	worst	9/1000

Figure 2. Health care expenditure as related to some health indicators.

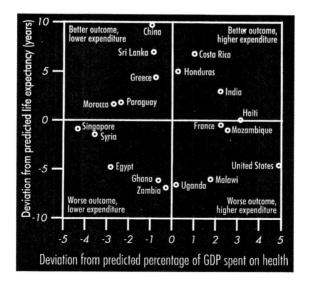

Figure 3. Life expectancy as related to health expenditure.

Several studies worldwide have demonstrated a close relationship between income increases and health improvements. Davey Smith and co-workers have established that the relation between health and socio-economic position is positive and progressive. (3 & 4)

However, it is also interesting to see that health improvements and income increases interact closely but act independently in response to other variables. (Fig 5). For example health of a population can improve without significant increases in GDP growth or per capita income. This depends upon how the increment is allocated at household or state level. For example, certain low and middle income countries show considerably better health indicators than other developing countries. Sri Lanka's citizens in 1991 had a life expectancy of 71 years, nearly the same as a lot of high income countries. (1)

Furthermore, health inequalities are universal in all societies, rich and poor. Inequality is therefore not only caused by deprivation in absolute terms, rather inequality is also a consequence of the distribution of social and economic advantages and the choices governments and people make. The increase in life expectancy over the 20th century has been

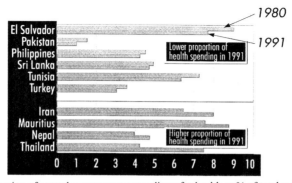

Figure 4. Proportion of central government expenditure for health as % of total public expenditure.

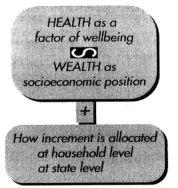

Figure 5. Relation between health and wealth.

greater in the upper social classes than the lower, nevertheless the improvement has been shared accross the range of socio-economic groups.

Probably there is also a synergy between different determinants of well-being (e.g. health, education) until a certain point of well-being is reached, but little information is available about this or about what happens after this point is reached. Therefore it can be concluded that wealth and economic growth are important for health but, in themselves, are insufficient to ensure people's well-being: appropriate use of the wealth and balanced choices which are made also count to a certain degree and are dependent upon individual, societal and political choices to be made.

2. SOME OF THE MAIN LESSONS TO BE LEARNED ON THE BASIS OF EXPERIENCES WITH HEALTH REFORMS AND HIV/AIDS

2.1. During the Last 10 years, Some of the Main Issues in the Health Reform Process Are:

- to make the health services more efficient to deal with disease
- to look for a biomedical cure of disease
- to redefine the roles of government, communities, individuals, public and private sector in organising and financing health services.

2.1.1. More Efficient Health Services. The worldwide restructuring of health services, and sometimes of social or sickness insurance systems, is focussing on economic viability of services in the framework of limited resources. This is true in developed and developing countries although the limits of the resources are of a very different scale for the two categories of countries. Moreover, redistribution of resources within and between countries is very difficult and clearly comes second place after efficiency of existing services has been ensured.

Better value of services for the money invested is commendable but surely not sufficient to improve health or well-being. A useful conclusion would be to keep the different objectives clearly separate. One objective is to more efficiently deal with health services while the other is to improve health, and both are not related in a simple and unilinear manner. Salutogenesis, complementing the pathogenesis model is only in its infancy.

2.1.2. Biomedical Cure. The other part of the response is related to the biomedical triumph model of western medicine, still heavily inclined to look for a biomedical cure, a magic bullet to cure and eradicate disease at individual and collective level. The cure model clearly has taken priority over care and prevention.

2.1.3. Redefinition of Roles. The roles of different players in organising and financing health services are being redefined. In this context, priority is presently given to decentralisation of services and privatisation. These are commendable methods to decrease the costs of services. However, what is the impact on health ? Clearly, more study is needed about the role of individual-oriented services versus what public health policies can achieve for health through different centralised or devolved models.

2.2. Some of the Lessons Learned from the HIV Epidemic

2.2.1. With HIV, care and cure had to go beyond the existing habits of giving a drug to kill the micro-organism. Therefore the HIV epidemic led us to start to deal better with the different entities of illness, disease, and sickness (Fig 6). The medical corps was reminded by people living with HIV that, before everything else, the person dealing with a disease needs support to bring harmony and to ensure that dignity and quality of life are a priority.

Although cure for HIV is not yet available for technical and/or economical reasons, care itself comes to the foreground as a basic right and a condition to ensure quality of life and dignity in the face of destiny.

2.2.2. Another experience shows that lower socio-economic status is correlated with shorter survival following HIV infection in the developing world and in some parts of the industrialised world (5). Factors such as social environment and others, external to the health care system as such, exert a major influence on HIV and health of the people (6 & 7). This recognition could trigger an evolution from a health care and health services policy to a health and quality of life policy as such. The case of HIV demonstrates also the importance of multifactorial elements influencing the acquisition, the transmission, the disease progression and the quality of life (Fig 7). The existing evolution in the medically oriented health care model had given little importance to those different aspects. The curative, biomedical model, believed since some decennia to enable us to get rid of infections and other diseases is now questioned by the infection itself.

2.2.3. HIV/AIDS also brings to the foreground the active role of individuals and societies to protect themselves and the community and to not wait passively for the medical corps to decide on people's lives.

> ❖ Illness: what the patient subjectively feels
> ❖ Disease: what the doctor biophysically relates to
> ❖ Sickness: how the patient is socioculturally perceived and cared for

Figure 6. Definitions of illness, disease, and sickness.

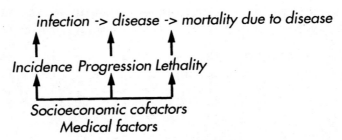

Figure 7. Socio-economic and cultural dimension of health.

In relation to the demand around HIV for individuals and communities to protect themselves, an obvious danger came about: "a social fracture". Some individuals with certain lifestyles becoming earlier infected in the industrialised countries than others could have started a further social fracture along the lines of already marginalised groups being perceived as populations at high risk to be discriminated and stigmatised. Active conscientisation must take place to counter the dangers of discrimination.

HIV demonstrated how stigmatisation and discrimination was a totally ineffective, inefficient and counter-productive measure and is not to be used as a public health intervention. **The only ethical public health response left was based on solidarity and care.**

2.2.4. Concerning the redefinition of the role of governments, public sector, private individuals, HIV has revealed a gap in a real culture of public health in relation to responsibilities of individuals, communities and governments. The example of blood infected with HIV in industrialised and developing countries should be a real learning process. Our biomedical and economic model has made it totally acceptable to wait for valid laboratory tests to be available and affordable before interventions to secure safety of blood become a priority. However, at that time we had another intervention already available, namely self-selection of donors related to clinical and lifestyle factors and based upon a responsibility of blood donors and governments. Some countries were earlier than others in taking the necessary measures. However, all were later than possibly could have been expected if the concept of health and well-being would have been seen as a social and collective issue rather than a biomedical issue not related to the community.

CONCLUSIONS

To a certain degree, wealth and health are inter-related but choices can be made which influence quality of life. Those choices are being made at different levels by governments and individuals.

The quality of life of human beings is achieved through a balance between health, knowledge, education, income and social interaction and infrastructure. In this contextual framework, people themselves do not pursue perfect health or education, but rather optimal health to achieve optimal quality of their lives.

People understand that if they try to maximise their health per se, it comes at a cost: for example sacrificing opportunities to travel, smoke and have sex.

Health reforms and HIV/AIDS have taught us major lessons. Health reforms have increased the focus on better management and cost containment, and HIV highlighted the interactions between socio-economic factors, disease and dignity and quality of life. Jointly, a major qualitative step forward could be made in the following years in the direction of dealing better with human capital and individual well-being worldwide.

Some of the main directions could be:

- to reach beyond a health care policy to a health policy that is itself an essential element of quality of life,
- to include the main parameters important for individuals. Going beyond the elusive concept of perfect health to a concept of optimal quality of life and dignity.
- reviewing the training and selection of health workers and the medical corps in this direction.

REFERENCES

1. World Development Report 1993. Investing in Health. Washington. Oxford University Press for the World Bank.
2. Human Development Report 1994. United Nations Development Programme (UNDP). New York - Oxford University Press. 1994.
3. Davey-Smith G, Bailet M, Blane D. The Black report on socio-economic inequalities in health 10 years on. BMJ 1990;301:373-376.
4. Davey-Smith G, Shyley MJ, Rose G. Magnitude and causes of socio-economic differentials in mortality: further evidence from the Whitehall study. Journal of Epidemiology and Public health 1990; 44:265-270.
5. Hogg RS, Strathdee SA, Craib KJP, O'Shaugnessy MV, Marloner JSG, Schecther MT. Lower socio-economic status and shorter survival following HIV infection. The Lancet 1994; 344: 1120-1124.
6. Fransen L, Whiteside A. The development - health connection: lessons for policy makers. Abstract submitted to the 23rd annual NCIH conference. Washington DC, June 1996.
7. Whiteside A, Fransen L. Assessing national and regional vulnerability and susceptibility to the HIV/AIDS epidemic. Abstract submitted to the XIth International Conference on AIDS. Vancouver, July 1996.

QUALITY OF LIFE

An Unsuitable Case for Measurement?

Sonta M. Hunt

Health Research
21 Teddington
Middlesex, England

The idea that there is an entity or construct known as "quality of life" has come have a wide currency and there are now a number of questionnaires which even purport to measure it. However, examination of the historical development and application of notions of quality of life show that it has been subjected to two kinds of cultural dominance.

First, the phrase "quality of life" has been largely appropriated by Medicine and Health Services Research both of which are embedded in Western empiricism, where objective, quantitative and verifiable data have precedence over the subjective, the qualitative and the phenomenological. This has had a profound effect, for example, on the form and content of questionnaires used to assess patients and to evaluate outcomes. Second, both the term "quality of life" and the measures used for its assessment grew out of a cultural background which was largely academic, middle-class, white and Anglo-Saxon. Questionnaires which originated in USA and, to a lesser extent, England have been deemed suitable for adaptation, translation and use in other countries. The ethnocentricity of this becomes apparent if we ask whether or not similar measures developed in China, Turkey or Nigeria would have been translated into English with the same enthusiasm and considered suitable for use in England, France, or the USA.

MEDICAL DOMINANCE

The mechanistic orientation of Western medicine has come to be accepted virtually world-wide. The underlying assumption is that human functioning and the manifestations of health and disease are more or less the same regardless of geography or culture. This assumption has also influenced constructions of quality of life, since they have been applied mainly within a medical setting. This perspective is reinforced by the fact that most people who work in the field of health measurement and quality of life assessment, when they travel to conferences in other countries, will probably meet individuals who, although from a different culture, are very similar to themselves. They share a common education and interests which are not at all representative of the diversity of inhabitants of their own country. Thus, there may appear to be a greater degree of cross-cultural uniformity than is actually the case. Many professional people are little acquainted with the variety of groups, ways of life and languages within their *own* country, never mind those of others.

A situation has arisen, therefore, where notions of quality of life are assumed to have the same universality as physiology, that is, to transcend culture and the meaning of "quality of life" has become firmly linked to health and disease. The coining of the term "health-related quality of life" even enabled old measures of health status to be presented, even promoted, in the guise of measures of quality of life, which they clearly were not. It is not possible to separate out effects due to health and those concomitant effects which are a consequence of changing patterns of finance, friendship, family life, responsibilities, expectations, occupations and so on. It is impossible to disentangle the strands of action and reaction, perception and misperception which are inextricably woven into the complex web of social and individual reality.

This dominance by a particular professional culture and the equating of health status with quality of life has reinforced the idea that quality of life is primarily about human functioning, for instance, optimal physical ability, the fulfilment of social roles and the declaration of certain psychological states. The content of questionnaires is not only reflective of professional notions of 'normality', it is also culturally biased. Thus a good "quality of life" becomes equated with optimal functioning defined within narrow confines of doubtful relevance to patients. Clearly, this is untenable and unethical. If we note that person A cannot walk as far as person B it is a perfectly reasonable statement on the comparison of physical capacity. However, to extrapolate from this to imply that, **therefore**, person B has a better **quality of life** not only discriminates against the physically disabled, the elderly and the chronically ill, but also imposes an arbitrary set of standards in relation to human experience which may well not apply outside the narrow confines of the professional and cultural world in which they were devised.

Human beings are reflective self conscious agents who interpret the world and events in a manner which is partly a consequence of social and cultural background and partly idiosyncratic. It is not the presence of symptoms or limitations of function which affect quality of life but rather the meaning and significance of them for individual patients. Thus, patients with an identical health status may experience a range of existential states from despair to happiness.

THE IMPORTANCE OF CONTEXT

The measurement of the so-called "quality of life" of individuals within medical settings has also isolated them from the cultural, social and material context within which they actually exist. Cross-culturally, even within some cultures, there is not always agreement about what constitutes a disease. How much more problematic is the definition for a construct such as "quality of life". Culture determines, to a great extent, which features of existence are regarded as part of the human condition and which may be regarded as indicative of illness. Sorrow, anxiety, angst, melancholy may all, for example, be regarded as perfectly reasonable responses to an unwelcome diagnosis and not necessarily evidence of the need for treatment or counselling.

The source of so-called "quality of life" questionnaires and their content do not and, indeed, cannot encompass the existential nature of quality of life and its various interpre-

22

QUALITY OF LIFE

Geographic and Cultural Differences

John Orley

Programme on Mental Health
Division of Mental Health and Prevention of Substance Abuse
World Health Organization
Geneva, Switzerland

The World Health Organization has, over the last ten years been working on the assessment of quality of life in health care settings. Some focused work in the last five years has resulted in the development of an instrument/questionnaire - the WHOQOL-100 - to assess Quality of Life (QOL)[1,2]. This instrument has been developed simultaneously in 14 countries around the world (e.g. France, India, Panama, Thailand, United States, Zimbabwe), representing very different cultural traditions.

At the start of the exercise, a group of investigators from most of the centres met to define what they considered to be QOL. It was defined as individuals' perception of their position in life in the context of the culture and value systems in which they live and in relation to their goals, expectations, standards and concerns. It is a broad ranging concept, incorporating in a complex way the person's physical health, psychological state, level of independence, social relationships, personal beliefs and relationship to salient features of the environment.

There are two key elements to this definition that dictate the form of the inquiry into a person's QOL. The first element is that it is subjective. It should reflect people's own perception of their position in life (and not a health professional's judgement on it). The WHOQOL does not attempt to determine people's attributes or possessions in an objective manner. For example, it does not assess level of income, neither absolute nor relative to those around them. It is concerned rather with their satisfaction with the income they have. Similarly, it does not ask as to how many hours people sleep but whether they are bothered by problems with sleep or not.

Secondly, QOL is defined for the purposes of the WHOQOL as multidimensional. Any assessment of QOL must explore a broad range of issues. It should not focus on a single issue, such as pain, (important though that may be for a particular individual), since such a focus cannot tell us what a person's overall QOL is like. If we wish to explore the QOL of people in pain, then we need to explore what it does to their social life, their psy-

Cancer, AIDS, and Quality of Life, edited by Levy *et al.*
Plenum Press, New York, 1997

chological life and their spiritual life and not just the effect on their physical functioning or mobility. Similarly, when exploring the QOL of people with AIDS, we need to look beyond the physical symptoms of the disease, to how it has affected their social life, their level of independence and other significant aspects of their life.

In addition to these two important aspects, the WHOQOL instrument explores positive aspects of life and is not a questionnaire focusing just on problems. QOL is about ease, not just the absence of disease.

The WHOQOL also differs from other commonly used QOL instruments in its contents. It includes items concerning personal beliefs (in a spiritual domain) and also items concerning how the environment affects health and health care. The environmental domain reflects the socio-economic indicators of QOL which have been used in the last 40 years or so, but it has turned these into subjective/satisfaction items. For example, a WHOQOL question asks about the satisfaction of the respondents with the condition of their living place, rather than the details of how spacious their living place is or what facilities are available in it. Other items within the environment domain in the WHOQOL have been chosen to reflect health related concerns, but the WHOQOL is not however, narrowly focused on health-related issues. It is an instrument with a broader sweep to its inquiry than most QOL measures and reflects more appropriately the concerns of most people around the world.

QOL is an alternative dimension of health outcome assessment, differing from others by its subjective approach. It does not invalidate relatively objective measures e.g. life expectancy or physical health parameters, but must not be confused with such objective measures. It would be expected that in general, the objective measures will be correlated with QOL, but it should not be assumed that this is the case in any individual.

Assessing QOL is not easy. In the absence of a consensus on what should constitute the core features of QOL, the measures tend to be indirect. Within the WHOQOL project, focus groups were run in different centres around the world to identify what were the features of life that were most important for the participants' QOL. In a way it must be realized that in order to explore quality, one has to explore the moderators of that quality. What the WHOQOL has done, is to take people back to fundamental moderators, rather than to focus on items that would be specific for an individual in a particular situation, or suffering from a particular disease. For example, someone under treatment for cancer, may lose all her hair. One can ask about her hair loss, but one can also ask how that hair loss itself affects QOL. It affects self-esteem, it affects bodily appearance, it might inhibit social contacts. If we continue to ask about how these things affect QOL, we come to a point at which these latter (e.g. social contacts) are identified as really fundamental to the respondents' quality of life, as opposed to those which may well be very serious, but which operate through their effects on the more fundamental moderators. It is at this fundamental level of inquiry that the WHOQOL is aimed. The WHOQOL therefore tends to be a generic instrument which can be used across a broad range of conditions and situations.

In making the focus group inquiry in the various participating centres, a number of very similar domains and subdomains (facets) which moderate quality of life, were identified. These seemed to be common to the groups in all of the geographically and culturally diverse centres. These broad domains can be summarized as the physical, the psychological, the social, the level of independence, the environment and a spiritual domain. This latter was insisted upon by the patients' focus groups despite a certain reluctance from clinicians. The items in this domain are phrased not so much in terms of religion, but with having a sense of meaning and purpose in life.

Surprisingly then, an agreement concerning the areas to be explored was obtained. The focus groups also suggested the ways that these areas could be explored, and surprisingly again, the questions identified by the various centres, for the instrument were very similar. Only in a few facets were major differences found. For example, self esteem was inquired into at most centres by asking questions about how subjects felt about themselves, but in South India in particular, the subjects wanted questions to inquire into how others felt about them (e.g. how satisfied are you with the respect that you get from others) and therefore this question was included. However, even in South India, which was the strongest proponent of such an approach, the questions (of respect from others) did not perform psychometrically as well as questions asking more directly about self respect in the pilot study. The same issue is arising again in our Chinese samples (not included in our first round) and will be explored again in terms of its importance for QOL in a Chinese population. This is not an unexpected issue. The very individualistic way that people identify themselves in the West has often been contrasted with the more social construction of identity in Eastern cultures.

Having defined and obtained a broad agreement about the areas of life that are important for determining its Quality; certain differences in the relative weightings of the importance of different facets between the various cultural groupings was found. We have yet to work out the significance of such differences, and whether they have to be taken account of in scoring. We explored this issue of importance by asking each subject in the pilot studies carried out at each centre, to rate the importance of each aspect of the facets that we had identified. In this way we discovered that there was almost universal agreement between our centres about those facets that were considered most important and those considered least important for QOL. Thus, performing activities of daily living, having energy, feeling healthy were all considered highly important. Sexual life was almost universally put at the bottom regarding its importance for QOL. It has to be said however that there was considerable variation in the rankings of those facets falling in the middle range.

It should however be noted that there were certain exceptions with respect to even the extreme positions. In Zimbabwe the facets "being able to get adequate health care" and "being able to get social help" were rated very highly, whereas this was not so in other centres. Indeed the item on "being able to get social help", ranked third from the top for Zimbabwe whereas it ranked 4th from bottom (of 41 items) in the global rankings. The spread of scores on importance ratings allows us to perform a hierarchical cluster analysis of centres regarding this issue. Many of the clusters obtained make sense - the North Indian with the South Indian (despite very different languages for the two centres - Hindi and Tamil). Another pair was Spain with Panama (in this case with language and cultural ties). Many of the West European influenced centres clustered together (France, Britain, United States, Australia - but with Israel and Croatia also).

In conclusion, it can be said that there seems to be broad agreement about the elements that constitute quality of life throughout the world and this can facilitate the development of an international measure of QOL. An instrument having the same core structure and content can be used to measure QOL across diverse cultures. But the relative importance attached to the individual facets may differ somewhat and this area is worth exploring further. The most useful and conceptually sound way of presenting QOL measurement results is also an area for further research. The WHOQOL Group intends to focus on these issues in the future.

REFERENCES

1. The WHOQOL Group. The World Health Organization Quality of Life Assessment (WHOQOL): Position Paper from the World Health Organization. Social Science and Medicine 1995:41:1403–1409.
2. Szabo S (on behalf of the WHOQOL Group). The World Health Organization Quality of Life (WHOQOL) Assessment Instrument. In: Spilker B, ed. Quality of Life and Pharmacoeconomics in Clinical Trials Second Edition. Philadelphia: Raven Publishers, 1996:355–362.

23

CANCER AND QUALITY OF LIFE

Social and Community Stakes

Patrice Pinell

INSERM U 158
Université René Descartes
Paris V

This paper intends to broach the question of the social and community stakes involved in quality of life in the field of cancer from the viewpoint of an historian who has studied changes in the ways this disease is dealt with. I will make no attempt to define what might or could be the "true" stakes involved in quality of life. Rather, my aim is much less ambitious, namely, to present certain contributions to the debate. These contributions, the result of looking at the past in a way that is more detached than engaged (to borrow from the concepts forged by Norbert Elias(1), aspire to bring about a better understanding of how and why quality of life can today be considered a stake for society.

Doctors in Ancient Greece already knew about cancer, yet before the 1960s no one spoke in terms of quality of life for cancer patients. The expression's commonplace definition was not accepted, nor, *a fortiori* was it accepted in its conceptual definition, which can be translated operationally by being included in questionnaires and used in "graphs." And so it is that for centuries, "quality of life" for people with cancer (and, generally speaking, victims of serious diseases) did not have enough meaning to become the object of social interests. Of course, this does not mean that patients were treated with total indifference, but rather that cancer was diagnosed when it was already well-advanced and it would inevitably lead to painful death. Suffering was clearly caused by the disease itself, but also by painful treatment, inflicting suffering that we know so little about alleviating.(2) Hence only a very black sense of humor could have thought in terms of "quality of life." If, starting in the 18th century, certain charitable energies were mobilized from time to time, it was mostly for those patients whose last days were spent in utter destitution and abandonment: the poor with cancer, who could find no place in the hospitals. Royal edicts enjoined the general hospitals to accept cancer patients, but hospital administrators often found a way to elude this obligation, sometimes offering small sums to patients who agreed to leave. The cause of disrepute for these patients was the stench of their sores, which aerist views at the time considered a source of infection for other patients. The small hospital for cancer patients in Reims, founded by Canon Godinot in the early 1740s, was the first and, for more than a century, the only institution where charitable concern for this kind of patient was translated into concrete terms. It endeavored to offer a place where the poor would be housed and fed, and where nurses would provide basic care (the doctor stopping by only very occasionally(3).

Built on similar premises, but this time deeply marked by the mystical tradition of heroic charity, the Association of the Ladies of Calvary was founded around 1850 in Lyons. This Catholic organization was made up of widows who had taken no religious vows. They paid to room and board and to have the honor of caring for cancer patients; they were tied to Calvary only by their love for God and the patients.(4) Being a widow was a mandatory condition to join, since "only the woman who has suffered and for whom the love of worldly things has disappeared is prepared to undertake this kind of work." The work involved caring exclusively for poor women suffering from ulcerous cancer; these women were often rejected by hospitals and hospices. (It was not until later that Calvary houses for men were set up.) Calvary houses were a community institution of sorts; they created a feminine micro-universe where patience combined with resignation, and faith with charity. An unusual feature of this micro-universe was its reversal of ordinary social relations: "Such is this most beautiful of all endeavors, where charity not only mixes and levels out the ranks, because it makes woman — who possesses birth, wealth, and for whom the world seems to reserve its delights — not only the companion, but the servant of the poor."(5)

The reference to the Calvary is more than an interesting detail. The association approached the first communitarian stakes related to "quality of life" for cancer patients, on two levels. For the women who devoted a part of their lives to this association, the stakes were personal. They had probably made this choice because they hoped to find consolation and healing of an "irreparable" wound in their lives. For the dominant classes, the stakes were social; the symbolic inversion of social relations as enacted by Calvary allowed the men of high society to portray themselves and perceive themselves in an enchanted vision, boasting of the goodness of their wealth, as they alone were able to care for the most unfortunate.(6)

The connection between the Calvary widows and the Ladies of the French Anti-Cancer League is evident if one considers that the first president of the Ladies' Central Committee, the Duchess of Uzäs, was also a Calvary widow.(7) Nevertheless, although the League denounced the sad lot of these incurables and made it one of its main battle themes, the strategies that guided the League's actions diverged from the communitarianism of the Calvary Association. While the Calvary created a self-enclosed world modelled on the convent, the League wanted to be a resolutely modern, "public health" association. While the Calvary was founded during an era when cancer was the paradigm of an incurable disease, the League was born — and this was its *raison d'être* — to combat a disease that public opinion had designated as a social scourge. This is precisely because cancer had become, under certain conditions, curable.(8) Let me explain: A disease is not elevated to the level of scourge unless one can consider (rightly or wrongly; this is not the question) that its effects are at least partially controllable. Since cancer eludes ordinary preventive methods, it could only be considered controllable from the time medicine achieved its first therapeutic successes. Thus the Anti-Cancer League was created to initiate and support the first cancer treatment centers, and its Ladies were mobilized to help in the care of patients. As a result they were quickly confronted, once again, with the problem of those who suffer from an incurable disease. Cancer treatment centers were expensive, but as part of the public hospital, they accepted and treated the poor. For practical reasons, patients who had been diagnosed as incurable were, as a matter of principle, not admitted. When treatment failed and a patient under the center's care passed into the category of incurables, he was supposed to be directed towards *ad hoc* facilities ("depository" run by the *Assistance publique* for incurable cancer patients, certain hospices that agree to accept them, the Calvary houses, etc). The job of finding a "bed" for these patients fell to the Ladies of the League in charge of "social service" at the center. For these ladies and young women of "good" social standing, the task proved to be earth-shattering. They discovered another world, that of overwhelming poverty and disease in the "promiscuity" of the slums. Their reaction was one of shock, indignation, often mixed with repulsion, and, at times, fascination.

The directors of the Anti-Cancer League attempted to use all their clout to see that the poor with incurable cancer would be cared for in treatment center annexes, in facilities designed for their specific needs. Given the indifference of nearly all the cancerologists and hospital administrators, they attempted, with the help of a few rare hospice doctors, to challenge the very relevance of the notion of incurability. They suggested replacing the opposition curable/incurable with a vision expressed in terms of remission. This would be an undetermined period of time during which the patient had to continue to receive medical care likely to prolong his life. Yet no heed was paid to the social question posed by incurable cancers until after World War II, when Nazi crimes against incurable patients were denounced. At this point, cancer treatment centers and public hospitals were charged with providing palliative care. The admission of patients to specialized centers marks a turning point, all the more remarkable because the function of the public hospital changed at precisely this moment. No longer devoted exclusively to a poor "clientele," the public hospital opened its doors to people from all social classes. The hospital became the place where the most modern medicine was practiced, ever more technical and ever more expensive.

The combination of the two phenomena (the admission of incurables, in a hospital for "all social classes") took effect before old practices had time to adapt. Thus emerged two new themes for criticism expressed in an especially vivid manner in cancerology. People spoke of the need to "humanize" hospitals and began to denounce using medical means to prolong the life of individuals who would otherwise die. The poor, who had no direct means to express their needs, found a "spokesman" in charity associations, which defined their interests for them. This time, criticism came from hospitalized patients themselves, or at least some of them. Within the dynamics of the May 1968 social movement, a certain spirit of protestation against the medical world began to develop. Groups of cancer patients with a critical frame of mind organized themselves; this was especially true of women with breast cancer. Yet these groups did not enjoy a great deal of continuity, and their relations with the League were not smooth. As a result, beginning in the 1960s, a variety of factors brought about a profound change in the charitable aspect of the association. Certain of these factors were related to general socio-cultural changes — a crisis in the recruitment of the Ladies who paid visits to patients, and the fact those who performed social work increasingly tended to be professionals. Other factors were more tied to changes in the fight against cancer. Cancer had become a "national cause" with one day every year devoted to fund-raising. The entire League concerned itself with collecting donations, both in terms of internal organization and in terms of its "message." This was the beginning of a process wherein the League began to accumulate considerable "wealth" and had the means to direct large sums of money in the field of cancerology. Although the League continued its efforts in terms of social assistance, its programs were increasingly carried out by professionals (paid and volunteer). The League became part of the cancer "establishment." Small associations of cancer patients had to work with such a League, and relations between the two often turned out to be conflictual. Indeed, relations grew strained as a result of the power at stake, with what could be perceived as one party being placed under the supervision of the other, but also because of divergent concepts about what associations should be (the charity tradition versus "self help" organizations). This tension was heightened by the "generation" and social gap separating directors of the League (wealthy class, high-placed civil servants) and the leaders of patients' associations (middle class individuals from intellectual professions). The latter had great difficulty establishing themselves and remaining financially autonomous, all the more so because of competition between the League and newcomer ARC,(9) which monopolized the public eye in the fight against cancer. Consequently, the existence of these patients' groups was often ephemeral, and their voices were heard only on occasion. Yet the social stakes regarding quality of life for cancer patients, as they appear today, would seem considerable, as have been the changes affecting patients' roles. Variations in treatment strategies and organizational and institutional methods of patient care have led to a situation wherein patients become an integrated part of the "assembly line" of medical activity; they act as "collaborators" of the medical staff... collaborators who are especially concerned with "company output" because their life is at stake, and because it determines the quality of their existence as well. This situation, which bestows a certain degree of autonomy on patients, is also rich in conflicting tensions. The patient plays a key role in medical care and is also the "object" of this care, at times assisting the medical staff, at times acting as a mostly "passive" patient. He may eventually experience treatment in a rather schizophrenic way.(8)

Given these conditions, it is easy to understand why patients organize themselves into associations. If this does not furnish an answer to the quality of life question, it at least provides a social space where the question can be discussed and benefit from an initial "treatment." It is also easy to understand why patients' organizations can be, along the lines of a union, a means for patients to defend their own interests, beginning with their interest in defining for themselves the relevant criteria used to assess "quality of life."

What remains to be seen is whether, by borrowing from and turning to AIDS associations for support, a patient-centered associative movement could establish itself in the world of the fight against cancer. It would need to break with a long history, deeply rooted in today's institutional reality. The question rests largely unanswered, and the historian is well aware that he who tries to predict the future is, scientifically-speaking, at best terribly naive, at worst a quack. The example of events in the United States shows that the "AIDS movement" can have significant impact on cancer patients' associations, yet the example cannot be directly transposed to France. The recent disqualification of a certain way of conceiving research support, and the fact that ARC has been (momentarily?) relegated to the sidelines, represent an element of profound readjustment in the sector concerned with the fight against cancer. How will this readjustment take place, with what repercussions on the emergence of a patient-centered movement, and by what means? Only time will tell!

REFERENCES

1. Elias N. Engagement et distanciation. Paris: Fayard, 1993.
2. Rey R. Histoire de la douleur. Paris: La Découverte, 1993.
3. Dr Pol Roger. L'hôpital pour cancérés. La lutte contre le cancer 1926;12:311-320.

4. Article on Calvaire, Dames du. In: Encyclopédie du catholicisme, hier, aujourd'hui et demain. Paris: Letouzey et Ané, t.II, 1954:400.

5. Roquain F. L'OEuvre des Dames du Calvaire, speech given December 10, 1904, at the Academy of Moral and Political Sciences. La Lutte contre le cancer 1924,3:207-213.

6. Pinell P. Naissance d'un fléau. Paris: Métailié, 1992.

7. Uzès (duchesse d'). Souvenirs de la Duchesse d'Uzès, née Mortemart. Paris: Plon, 1939.

8. Pinell P. *op. cit.*

9. ARC = *Association pour la recherche contre le cancer* (Association for Research Against Cancer)

24

THE HIV/AIDS EPIDEMIC IN DEVELOPING COUNTRIES

The Dilemma of Quality of Life vs Quality of Care

Ibrahim M. Shoaib

Professor of Public Health
Tanta University
Faculty of Medicine
Egypt

INTRODUCTION

As the number of HIV-infected persons approaches 20 million world-wide and with more than 4.5 million AIDS cases by late 1995, the scientific community is still years away from finding an effective cure or preventive measures to curb the devastating spread of the HIV pandemic.

In most developing countries; especially those in sub-Saharan Africa, the home of more than 11 million HIV infections (55% of the world total) and more than 3 million AIDS cases (70.7% of the world total); the great majority of HIV/AIDS patients have no access to a decent and a universally-acceptable minimum standard of medical care and support for themselves and their families. They have already experienced the increasing health, social and economic burden of the epidemic, suffered from the negative consequences of the imposed Structural Adjustment Policies (SAPs) and have struggled for socio-political stability after decades of bitter war-strifes, tribal conflicts, civil injustices and apartheid. They face complex and difficult problems of rising debts, frequent famines, market depression and refugees. These sub-Saharan countries and most other developing countries will not be able to provide a decent and proper medical care and socio-psychological support to the rising numbers of HIV/AIDS.

QUALITY OF LIFE

Poverty, with all its associated social evils and ill-health, remains the formidable challenge facing most of the developing countries toward realizing their national development and progress. In these countries, the number of poor people has been rising since the

Cancer, AIDS, and Quality of Life, edited by Levy *et al.*
Plenum Press, New York, 1997

1980s, with per capita income declining from $563 annually in 1980 to $485 annually in 1992. More than one billion people in developing countries live in absolute poverty, more than 100 million people are overtly unemployed, more than one billion adults are illiterate, and over 300 million children do not go to schools. More than 1.3 billion people lack access to safe drinking water and more than 1.8 billion are deprived from sanitary and basic health services. More often than not, poor people marginalized and excluded from access to basic social and health services and are therefore under-nourished, in bad health and poorly educated. Over 13 million children under the age of 5 years die annually in developing countries, essentially from preventable diseases.

The present ongoing efforts by the WHO for the development of an International Assessment Instrument of quality of life (WHOQOL) is based on the WHO definition of quality of life as "an individual's perception of his/her position in life in the context of the culture and value systems in which he/she lives, and in relation to his/her goals, expectations, standards and concerns". This definition is inseparable from the other WHO's definition of health as "a state of physical, mental and social well-being, not merely the absence of disease or infirmity". With prevailing poverty in developing countries and wide-spread global inequity between the North and the South, it is very hard to imagine that the proposed WHOQOL can be fairly and objectively applied with regard to completely different patterns and systems of health and disease in completely different and separate two worlds. HIV/AIDS, in addition to being a fetal disease, has significant negative impact on health, social, psychological, economic civil and legal aspects of life, which actually constitute the main domains of the individual's quality of life. For a person in the prime of life being diagnosed as having an incurable and terminal illness is a devastating experience. This feet demands tremendous reserves of courage, patience and determination. It also requires a great deal of care and support from government services, non-government organizations (NGO), private sectors, employers, local communities, friends and family.

QUALITY OF CARE

Finance and trained professionals available affect the quality of care given to HIV/AIDS patients and their families and hence their quality of life. Most people believe that human life is virtually priceless and public health professionals would be unwise to put a monetary value on human life. However, all decisions regarding resource allocation to health and medical care services carry with them an implicit valuation of life. Today, all over the world, there are competing for limited resources, conflict over their uses (e.g. health vs education vs social welfare vs defense), conflict within the health sector itself (e.g. prevention vs cure, palliative vs curative, alternative schemes of long-term care and support), and conflict over the use of scarce public and even private funds for so many somewhat expensive health services for terminally ill and/or handicapped people (e.g. cancer, HIV/AIDS patients). In the face of this decisions, the great majority of people especially in developing countries, are facing death because of lack of adequate basic sanitary and health services (e.g. safe-drinking water, latrines, immunization, Oral Rehydration Solution (ORS), Maternal and Child Health Services (MCH), Family Planning (FP) and Sexually Transmitted Diseases (STDs) treatment).

Developing countries especially those in the sub-Saharan Africa, are faced with pressing challenges of providing long-term care and support, for decades to come, to increasing numbers of frequently and/or terminally ill and handicapped HIV/AIDS patients and their families. The mission seems impossible, unless there is a quick and highly concerted and coordinated international effort to ameliorates the prevailing poverty in the South and bridge the widening gap of social and economic inequities between the North and the South. Without such effort, developing countries will be heading toward a bleak future for the following reasons:

1. The Unique Characteristics of HIV/AIDS Illness

Not like any other disease in the history of mankind, the medico-scientific community has to face new and exceptional challenges of the global HIV/AIDS epidemic characterized by:

a. A long incubation period (IP) of HIV infection, which may extend to 10 years. During this period, the HIV-infected person can transmit the virus to other people through sexual contact, blood and other body fluids and the infected mother to her baby during pregnancy, labor and after labor. This fact also means that the actual numbers of HIV-infected people at any given time can not be accurately determined and can remain hidden and unknown for several years.

b. HIV infection is permanent and almost always ends in AIDS and death. There is neither a cure for a preventive vaccine.

c. The victims of HIV infection are primarily sexually active adolescents and young adults of both sexes i.e. the fittest and productive sector of the population, and hence it has been called "The killer of the Fittest". The huge burden of excessively losing this sector of the population is already being experienced in many national sectors-whether economic, services, education or health and at all levels in many of the developing countries especially in sub-Saharan Africa.

d. HIV infection lays the ground for the emergence and spread of many dangerous diseases which were thought to have been placed under control (e.g. tuberculosis (TB), diarrhoeal diseases, malaria).

e. HIV/AIDS epidemic in developing countries could easily reverse health gains and triumphs achieved in the 1970s and early 1980s, following decades of huge national and international investments and efforts, especially in areas of maternal and child health, infectious diseases control and TB control.

2. Obstacles to Long-Term Medical Care and Support

Already suffering from scarce health and medical resources, over-stretched and inadequate health services and inability to realize their national development plans in areas of health and social welfare, most developing countries are facing the challenges of overcoming difficult obstacles for providing an adequate and proper long-term medical care and support to increasing numbers of HIV/AIDS patients and their families. These obstacles include:

a. Not enough drugs or no drugs at all to treat medical conditions associated with HIV/AIDS e.g. anti-fungal and anti-tuberculous drugs and the problem of dealing with the emergence of multiple drug resistant strains of TB. In addition, most developing countries would not dream of using any of the prohibitively expensive anti-retroviral drugs which constitute the back-bone therapy for HIV/AIDS patients in industrialized countries.

    b. Insufficient numbers of properly trained health professionals capable of coping with unique health, social and psychological needs of frequently ill, handicapped and/or dying young adults and adult patients.

    c. Wide-spread discrimination, stigmatization and prejudice toward people known or believed to have HIV/AIDS and the need for civil and legal protection as regard to specific rights such as securing employment, pensions, health care, medical confidentiality, education freedom of travel and women's and children's right to inherit property. Discrimination and prejudice and related loss of human rights and dignity further increase the vulnerability to HIV/AIDS.

    d. The prevailing public ignorance about the nature of HIV/AIDS and the unrealistic public attitudes, beliefs and feelings toward the epidemic.

    e. The wide-spread play down seriousness of the HIV/AIDS problem by many governments, and the delays in policy after more than 14 years from the start of the epidemic.

    f. The great diversity of un-coordinated activities and initiatives in providing medical care and support to HIV/AIDS patients and their families which lack a universally acceptable minimum standard of quality care guidelines.

Even with substantial injections of financial, physical and human resources, it will become increasingly difficult for developing countries especially those in sub-Saharan Africa, to meet the needs of the rising numbers of HIV/AIDS patients and their families without compromising the basic health and social care provision to those who are not infected. Painful and difficult decisions have to be made on how scarce health resources should be allocated between prevention and treatment of HIV/AIDS conditions and other diseases.

Action is urgently needed. The problem of poverty and the global inequity must not be ignored. It sooner or later affects every one. It travels across borders without passport in the form of diseases, drugs, pollution, migration, political instability and terrorism. It is only where rights and responsibilities within the global society of nations and individuals are fully respected, assumed and shared, can poverty, inequity and HIV/AIDS pandemic be addressed with success.

REFERENCES

1. Khor, M. Structural adjustment degrades. In UNEP Magazine "Our Planet", 1995, Vol. 7, No. 1, p. 20.
2. O'Donahue,. The impact of HIV/AIDS on hospitals and health services: Is AIDS a development issue?. UK NGO AIDS Consortium for the Third World, London, 1990.
3. Orley, J. and Kuyken W. Quality of life assessment: International perspectives. Springer Verlag, Berlin, New York, 1993.
4. The Panos Institute. Panos Dossier: The hidden cost of AIDS. Panos Publ. Limited, London, Paris, Washington, 1992.
5. WHO. Cumulative infection approach 20 million. In Global AIDSNEWS Newsletter of WHO/GPA, Geneva, 1995, No. 3/4.

25

QUALITY OF LIFE

Some Implications of the Advances in Human Genome Research

Paul A. Marks

Memorial Sloan-Kettering Cancer Center
New York, New York 10021

CONTEXT

This symposium, "Cancer, AIDS and Quality of Life," has focused on the quality of life issues of individuals and societies in managing the challenges facing patients with AIDS or with advanced cancers. There is a clear and urgent need to develop better programs and generate more financial resources for appropriate supportive care that can be provided to improve the quality of life for so many in the late stages of these diseases (1).

In the context of the entire challenge that cancers and AIDS represent, a distinction should be made between these afflictions. Essentially fifty percent of all cancers (not including skin and cervical cancers which should be over ninety-five percent curable) can be controlled or cured today, while AIDS remains an incurable disease. Without diminishing the importance of the quality of life issues that are particular to the incurable stages of these diseases, perhaps the most important contribution we can make to the quality of life of individuals at risk for cancer is to emphasize the importance of prevention and early detection (when cancers are most likely to be cured).

It is in this context that I will briefly consider the impact that advances in human genome research will increasingly have on the "quality of life" of almost all of us. Let us examine, albeit briefly, two aspects of genetic research; 1) the impact of discovery of genes that place individuals at an increased risk for cancer, and 2) gene discovery that is changing the approach to new drug development.

PREDICTIVE TESTING FOR CANCER BY GENE TESTING

Predictive testing by identifying individuals at hereditary risk for cancer or other disease at a clinically presymptomatic stage and intervening to prevent or effectively treat the disorders is the great promise that such an approach holds for us today. This approach

Cancer, AIDS, and Quality of Life, edited by Levy *et al.*
Plenum Press, New York, 1997

could improve the quality of life for many—substantially reducing human suffering and the economic burden of these diseases. On the other hand, there are many issues to be addressed before we can effectively realize the benefits of these advances in gene research. Indeed, it is likely that as we go forward with genetic testing, there is the potential for adversely affecting the quality of life for some people by causing increased anxiety, depression, grief and/or economic pain. There are many reasons that this may occur.

As examples, there is the need to develop accurate diagnostic tests for the risk gene(s), professional counseling services as to the pros and cons of testing for an individual and his/her family must be developed and offered, and effective interventions to prevent or treat the disease must be available. At the present time, we are limited in each of these areas.

IDENTIFYING GENES THAT INCREASE RISK FOR CANCER

Genetic research is identifying genes which are associated with an increased risk for one or another cancer. Tests for a number of such genes are already available and we can anticipate that many more will be discovered over the next few years. There are issues related to reliability of the tests, the validity of "risk" assessments, guidelines for who should be tested, and the economies of testing to mention a few up-front questions related to the applications of such gene testing to clinical practice.

Today, we can relatively easily identify individuals at risk for certain genetically determined diseases which are associated with a mutation in a single gene. An example of such a disease whose outcome can be predicted with considerable accuracy is Huntington's Disease, a fatal and incurable neurodegenerative disease that affects around 1 in 20,000 of the European population during mid-life. Unfortunately, there is not yet any intervention to prevent or effectively treat this disease. Another is cystic fibrosis (CF) which is caused by mutations in a relatively large gene. Cystic fibrosis affects approximately 1 in 12,500 of the Caucasian populations in North America and Northern Europe. The testing for a specific defect in the CF gene is more complicated. Seventy percent of the patients with cystic fibrosis carry a particular known mutation in the gene that encodes the protein responsible for the disorder. A negative test for this mutation does not guarantee freedom from the disease because a potential sufferer of cystic fibrosis could be carrying any one of 500 known mutations within the same relatively large gene that can be associated with the disease and go undetected by the test.

Genes have been identified which place individuals at increased risk for breast cancer, colon cancer and a number of other less common cancers. In the case of breast cancer, at least two genes, BRCA1 and BRCA2, have been identified which are associated with an increased risk for breast cancer. In the case of colon cancer, mutations in any of five separate genes are known to increase an individual's risk to develop colon cancer. In both of these examples, the absence of such mutations does not necessarily mean that the person who has been screened will not develop either disease.

Take breast cancer, 1 in 10 women living in western societies are likely to develop this disease by the age of 85 and 25% of these sufferers will die from the disease. Only about 5% of breast cancers seem to be strongly hereditary. Mutations in the two known susceptibility genes, BRCA1 and BRCA2, appear to account for 80% of these hereditary cases, i.e., 80% of the 5% of cases are only about 4% of all patients who develop breast cancer. The mutation clearly requires communicating the fact that genetic testing for BRCA1 and BRCA2 will be of little value to some women even though they are predisposed to the cancer and even of less value for about 95% of women in whom breast cancer will develop that is not associated with a strong hereditary predisposition (2,3).

EMOTIONAL AND BEHAVIORAL CONCERNS WITH RESPECT TO GENETIC TESTING

As genetic testing for susceptibility to cancer becomes widely available, cancer-care providers will become more involved in counseling patients about cancer risk and the meaning of genetic test results. It is already clear from numerous studies (2–9) that we can anticipate substantial emotional and behavioral responses to the disclosure of genetic status. These responses will differ in different individuals, but include anxiety, depression and guilt. These responses have the potential to affect functional health status. For example, it has been reported that as many as 30% of women who know themselves to be at risk for breast cancer suffer a functional impairment due to concerns about their personal risk status. These findings underscore the importance of recognizing the possible impact of predictive genetic testing on many aspects of the quality of life.

There is, of course, another side to predictive genetic testing. Predictive testing can alleviate fear of being at risk; early diagnosis can increase the chances for effective prevention or therapy. It will be unfortunate if we cannot realize these advantages because we do not adequately address the potential negatives of predictive testing. This requires a great deal of further research at the genetic level (tests for genes), at the counseling level (developing appropriate guidelines for counseling) and, perhaps most importantly, at the intervention level (preventive and therapeutic modalities).

POTENTIAL UNFAIR USES OF GENETIC INFORMATION

There are another set of challenges in the application of genetic testing that affect the quality of life. One can speculate on a range of situations in which personal genetic information can be used unfairly. These include such areas as employment, life, health and disability insurance, automobile insurance, adoption, dental licensure, qualification for mortgage, admission to medical school, and admission to various health care plans. There will be an increasing number of genes for which we will be able to test that predispose individuals to diseases such as cancers, heart disease, diabetes, arthritis, etc. While it is easy to exaggerate both our current ability and the speed with which these genetic tests are likely to become available, one cannot overemphasize what remains to be done in understanding not only how different gene defects may lead to a particular disease, but also how valid are the risk estimates related to the presence of a particular gene and how to proceed with testing in clinical practice. For certain abnormal genes related to cancer or other diseases, it may require years of follow-up and careful analytical studies to establish the risk implications and guidelines for the effective use of the test for a particular gene(s). It may be presumed that as we gain more experience with genetic tests and as more genetic tests are developed, we will gain experience on how to most effectively apply these tests to the benefit of individuals. At present, however, we are not in that situation and in the opinion of many, regulation in the use of genetic information is required. Indeed, in an editorial in *Nature* (2), it was suggested that "a short and sharp moratorium on the use of genetic information by insurers, combined with fierce public debate followed by initial regulations that are deliberately overcautious and a subsequent period of liberalization, as more becomes known of both the real and hypothetical dangers posed" to the quality of life may be a reasonable public policy approach to these issues.

At present, the situation regarding legislation related to the use of genetic information is a mixed bag. In the United Kingdom, Germany, Japan, Italy, Spain and Portugal, there are no laws governing the use by insurance companies of the results of genetic tests. In France and the Netherlands there is a moratorium, that is a temporary prohibition, on the use of genetic information by insurance companies. In the United States, ten states prohibit genetic testing and the use of genetic information for health insurance purposes.

Despite the possible downside to predictive testing, it is clear that over the next several years a number of tests will become available to the general public for identifying genes that place individuals at an increased risk for cancer and other diseases. Indeed, there are companies that already market such tests. Among the issues raised by the availability of these tests including: who should be offered the tests and under what conditions? While there is no consensus with respect to these questions, it seems wise that the tests currently available, including those for breast and colon cancer, be offered under strict protocol research studies so that much more can be learned about the validity of data of risk prediction, how to effectively counsel individuals prior to and following testing, about the consequences of receiving information that one is at risk or that one is not at risk, and the costs of testing. The fact is that problems of unfair genetic discrimination and its impact on the quality of life must be evaluated by projecting into a future full of uncertainty. Such uncertainty should not and, undoubtedly, will not, per se, delay genetic research. The fact is that the "genetic revolution" is and will have a growing impact on the quality of life of many individuals in our society. It is essential we address the issues raised as best we can, with the hope that as we learn more, we will be able to better address them.

GENE DISCOVERY AND DRUG DISCOVERY

The quality of life has increasingly been affected by the effectiveness of preventive and therapeutic interventions in sustaining health and ameliorating the consequences of disease. Remarkable progress has been made over the years in the prevention of many diseases with vaccinations such as poliomyelitis, small pox, measles, rubella, yellow fever, and others which were devastating factors in undermining the quality of life. Substantial advances have been made in the control of bacterial infections, cardiovascular diseases, many cancers and other major chronic ailments. With all these advances, we have had relatively little impact on a number of diseases, particularly those of viral origin such as AIDS, ebola and influenza, to mention but a few. Certain parasite diseases, such as malaria, remain a major threat in vast parts of the world. Definitive therapy is also not at hand for metastatic cancers, chronic arthritis, diabetes mellitus, Alzheimer's, neurodegenerative diseases, atherosclerosis, and other ailments that now are so-called chronic diseases. The advances in defining the human genome and, in particular, identifying the role that specific genes play in the control of growth and differentiation of cells and organisms, have great promise for providing direct approaches to new therapeutic interventions by identifying new targets for effective approaches to the cure or control of the diseases. Indeed, defining the human genome and understanding the biological role of specific genes is fundamentally changing the approach to drug discovery. Increasingly, medicine will be moving from a paradigm of diagnose and treat to one of predict and prevent. You have only to follow the reports in the daily media to feel the excitement and potential of genomic research.

Literally hundreds of companies and thousands of research laboratories in academic institutions and in industry are pursuing research to identify genes, discover their biological function and develop new targets for drugs in areas as diverse as osteoporosis, high blood pressure, diabetes, Alzheimer's disease, breast cancer, colon cancer, prostate cancer, obesity and muscular disorders, and many others.

Gene research can impact drug discovery in several ways. The most direct and, probably the least important over the long run, is the direct replacement of a defective or absent gene through gene therapy. Another approach is to directly affect the expression or regulation of the defective gene in such a way as to ameliorate the disease. These therapeutic approaches may be particularly useful in so-called monogenetic diseases. These are diseases in which a single abnormal gene is identified as the basis of the development of the disease such as is the case in Huntington's disease, cystic fibrosis, or Duchenne's Muscular Dystrophy. Another approach is to block the expression of the defective gene using constructs of "antisense" which have the opposite but exact base structure of the defective gene and will combine with the defective gene and block its activity so as to prevent its damaging effect. To date, there has been no successful development of gene therapy in human subjects. It remains a major conceptual as well as practical challenge.

What seems more promising, is to identify appropriate targets through genetic research for the development of new chemicals of therapeutic value. It is estimated that there are approximately 100,000 functioning genes in a human subject and that we understand the function of only about on 10% of these genes. Understanding the function of the gene is critical to developing targets for possible chemicals that can block or activate, depending on the desired result, the effects of a gene that is the cause of a disease. The potential of this new approach to drug discovery is very exciting and clearly will impact the quality of life across the spectrum of many acute (e.g., viral diseases) and chronic (e.g., metastatic cancers) diseases for which there is now no effective therapeutic intervention.

CONCLUSIONS

The ongoing "revolution" in biomedical research, specifically in human genome research, will have a profound impact on the quality of life. In this brief presentation, we have identified two major areas: 1) predictive testing based on identifying individuals with genes that increase risk for disease; and 2) development of new approaches to drug discovery based on targets identified through the discovery of genes that may be the basis of disease.

Predictive genetic testing has the potential to markedly improve the quality of life through enhancing the possibility for disease prevention and health maintenance, as well as, the detection of disease early when it is most curable. On the other hand, it has the potential for a negative effects by identifying an individual at increased risk for disease without having an effective intervention to prevent or cure the disease and by exposing the individual to adverse discrimination which may be devastating. One cannot stop, nor should one want to stop, the progress in human genome research. Rather, we must focus a great deal of attention on how to apply the products of this research to improve the quality of life.

REFERENCES

1. Support Principal Investigators. A controlled trial to improve care for seriously ill hospitalized patients. Journal of the American Medical Association 1995:274:1591–1598.

2. Editorial. Whose right to genetic knowledge? Nature 1996:379:379.
3. Massod E. Gene test: Who benefits from risk? Nature 1996:379:389–392.0
4. Lerman C, Croyle RT. Emotional and behavioral responses to genetic testing for susceptibility to cancer? Oncology 1996:10:191–199.
5. Baker SG, Freedman LS. Potential impact of genetic testing on cancer prevention trials using breast cancer as an example. Journal of the National Cancer Institute 1995:87:1137–1144.
6. Billings PR, Kohn MA, deCuevas M, Beckwith J, Alper JS, Natowicz, MR. Discrimination as a consequence of genetic testing. American Journal of Human Genetics 1992:50:476–482.
7. Natowicz MR. Genetic discrimination and the law. American Journal of Human Genetics 1992:50:465–475.
8. Allen W, Ostrer H. Anticipating unfair uses of genetic information. Invited Editorial, American Journal of Human Genetics 1993:53:16–21.
9. Brown ML, Kessler LG. The use of gene tests to detect hereditary predisposition to cancer: Economic consideration. Journal of the National Cancer Institute 1995:87:1131–1136.

QUALITY OF LIFE IN CANCER AND AIDS

An Industry Perspective

Stephen K. Carter

Research and Development
Boehringer Ingelheim Pharmaceuticals, Inc.
Ridgefield, Connecticut

The goal of clinical research in cancer and AIDS is either curative or palliative in intent. In cancer cure is defined as long term disease free survival which is comparable to the survival of individuals without the disease. In cancer cure is possible, with optimal therapy, in nearly half the patients. For the other half in cancer and for all individuals with AIDS palliation is the goal. Palliation can be defined as the alleviation of symptoms and/or prolongation of survival. Inherent in all of this is the assumption that cure and palliation will have a positive impact on quality of life.

In cancer and AIDS the concept of palliation is often denigrated. This may result from disappointment that cure is not being achieved with resultant downgrading of short term survival prolongation. Another contributing factor may be the perceived side effects of the therapies and the assumption that quality of life will not be meaningfully improved with short term (months to years) survival gains. What is often overlooked is that many major diseases are not cured e.g., diabetes, hypertension, arteriosclerotic heart disease, and that palliation is all that is achieved with treatment. It would be interesting to compare the relative survival of an individual newly diagnosed with congestive heart failure with one newly diagnosed with AIDS. In both scenarios palliation of symptoms with prolongation of survival is the therapeutic goal and yet only in AIDS would you have to deal with a philosophy of nihilism which would question whether any therapy is worthwhile.

Improving the quality of life of individuals with cancer or AIDS can only occur through clinical research improving the cure rates or the palliative potential. In these diseases however those who study quality of life often tend to focus on scenarios where therapeutic results are assumed to be poor or on terminal care. As important as these areas may be, disease free survival should be assumed to be a therapeutic result which will significantly enhance quality of life.

It will be new therapies therefore that will offer the greater hope of improving quality of life. The research based pharmaceutical industry is dedicated to finding new therapies for cancer and AIDS. While government agencies and academia receive the lions

Cancer, AIDS, and Quality of Life, edited by Levy *et al.*
Plenum Press, New York, 1997

share of publicity, it is the pharmaceutical industry which has discovered the great majority of new drugs and it is the industry that has developed all of them for widespread usage through approval of commercial sale by regulatory agencies. A new therapy will not improve quality of life unless it is available to all who may benefit from it. It will not be widely available until it is approved for commercial sale. It is the incentives of commercial sale that allow the pharmaceutical industry to spend billions on the research and development of new drugs for major killers such as cancer or AIDS. It costs over 300 million dollars and takes approximately ten years to successfully develop a drug, and many drugs fail to be successfully developed.

The pharmaceutical industry utilizes the tools and the methodology of clinical research to develop a new drug. This involves sequential clinical trials that are conceptually classified as phase I, II or III. All three phases are therapeutic intent trials in patients with the disease. Phase I involves dose determination and side effect evaluation. Phase II involves evaluation of the efficacy potential and a predicting of the ultimate therapeutic index. Phase III trials are large scale trials, usually controlled, to demonstrate an efficacy and safety profile that will satisfy the regulatory requirements for commercial scale. In cancer and AIDS the requirements are different in different parts of the world and therefore global development is an expensive and labor intensive challenge.

The pharmaceutical industry has three perspectives on clinical research which are conceptually important to separate even though they overlap to some degree. The traditional research perspective involves hypothesis testing with the goal of adding meaningfully to the research database. The patient care perspective focuses on how the result in the population of the clinical trial extrapolates to individual patient care. Put another way, how would a physician faced with a patient in their clinic or office change his or her therapeutic approach based on the trial results. Implicit in this is a population based extrapolation of the therapeutic index of a therapy to a single patient. Physicians will modulate this by their understanding of the entire database and their past clinical experience. The bottom line will be to improve the quality of life of the patient by either cure or palliation.

The regulatory perspective involves meeting the regulatory criteria for efficacy and safety so as to achieve widespread availability. This involves a dossier of results from multiple clinical trials with the aim of achieving a broad population based extrapolation of the therapeutic index from the dossier to a regulatory agency approved recommendation of how a physician should use the drug in approaching new individual patients.

Within the framework of these clinical trial perspectives there exists a range of efficacy criteria in AIDS and cancer. The most controversial of these are the surrogate markers. In cancer this is the objective response. In AIDS it is either the CD4 lymphocyte count, or the viral load which can be measured by several different techniques. These are controversial because there is lack of agreement and how well they predict for the clinical endpoints of overall and disease free survival which are deemed to be the most important and reliable indicators for the bottom line of improving or sustaining quality of life. While quality of life is the ultimate goal its measurement as an efficacy criteria is not established. This is the case because the scales which attempt to measure quality of life are designed to objectify the subjective. There is no one scale considered to be validated to the point where they could be basis of a regulatory decision or a hypothesis validation. At this time quality of life is considered an ancillary efficacy evaluation to enhance the interpretation of surrogate marker and clinical endpoint data.

The controversies about the surrogate markers prediction for clinical endpoints tends to obscure some important realities. One of these realities is that drug development would not be possible in AIDS or cancer without them. All phase I and II trials utilize surrogate markers. Clinical endpoints in these trials would not be feasible and if required would essentially end drug development as we know it. Every drug currently used to treat cancer or AIDS was first discovered to be efficacious utilizing surrogate markers. It can therefore be said that every drug on the market for both diseases is a true positive for the surrogate marker prediction of efficacy. If one looked at the history of drug development in these disease, the false positives have not been many. What we do not know anything about is the false negative rate. The fact remains however that these surrogate markers have a better track record than many are willing to give them credit for.

Another aspect of surrogate markers is that they are the basis of most of the individual patient care decisions. In HIV a physician monitors the CD4 count and both starts, stops and changes therapy based on their fluctuations. A cancer physician will continue to treat if the tumor is shrinking or remains stable, and will stop and/or change them if the tumor is enlarging. All of these decisions will be modulated by the physician and the patient continuously evaluating quality of life although it is rarely undertaken utilizing formal scales.

Surrogate markers are well established and non controversial in many chronic diseases in which cure is not a therapeutic reality. These surrogate markers include: 1) blood pressure lowering in hypertension; 2) lipid lowering in cardiovascular diseases; 3) blood sugar lowering in diabetics and; 4) pulmonary function tests in respiratory diseases.

The evaluation of quality of life utilizing objectifying scales is increasing within clinical research. Since quality of life is the bottom line for a patient approaching treatment, this is logical. There exist however a range of challenges to be met. The first is the development of a standardized methodology that will be used by a wide range of investigators so that a meaningful database can be built up. This database will allow more secure evaluation of a new result. A second challenge will be to correlate quality of life results with the standard efficacy criteria such as surrogate markers and clinical endpoints. This will entail how to utilize the results in the short term decision making of early (phase I-II) drug development trials and in the patient care decisions of when to stop, start and switch therapy. A third challenge which overlaps with the first two is how to integrate quality of life into the three perspectives of clinical research i.e., research, patient care and regulatory.

QUALITY OF LIFE, VALUE, AND PRICE IN MEDICINES TO TREAT SERIOUS DISEASE

Robert E. Cawthorn

Rhone-Poulenc Rorer Inc.
500 Arcola Rd.
PO Box 1200
Collegeville, Pennsylvania 19246-0107

INTRODUCTION

There are many reasons for attempting to measure the quality of life impact of medicines on diseases such as cancer and AIDS. For the doctor it provides evidence of how well a patient is responding to treatment; for patients they become involved in their treatment and feel able to influence it. But what does it do for measuring the economics of that treatment?

When quality of life measurements show that, because of treatment, there has been substantial improvement, it can provide reassurance for purchasers that money is being spent wisely. But should these data move beyond financial reassurance and towards resource allocation? For pharmaceuticals, this is important because resource allocation affects the price and the volume of drug used.

Today I will examine three of the issues involved in the measurement of quality of life in the pharmaceutical treatment of serious disease. These are the accuracy and quality of our quality of life measures; the value of these measures in aiding resource allocation in well satisfied disease areas and in unsatisfied ones; and to raise a cautionary note about the use such measurement could be put to.

1. HOW GOOD ARE OUR QUALITY OF LIFE MEASURES?

Health systems always have to compare apples with oranges in resource allocation. They have to choose between treatment options within a therapy area, and between therapy areas themselves. And they frequently have to do so without the sort of data which we in business take for granted. Do quality of life data provide a common ground for judging the value gained from each of these treatment options? It has been said that a cynic is someone who knows the price of everything and the value of nothing. Do quality of life

Cancer, AIDS, and Quality of Life, edited by Levy *et al.*
Plenum Press, New York, 1997

data overcome what by this definition could be defined as the "cynicism" of many health systems?

The Evaluation of Quality of Life

We have come a long way from the early cost-benefit assessments, which simply weighted costs against healthcare savings. The measurement of the number of years of extra life gained is an important tool, but it has an obvious fundamental deficiency. If life is extended by, say, three years and if these years are spent in greater pain and in a bed-ridden condition, the value of these extra years is small. Or so the professional could think. But what if your daughter or granddaughter was getting married, or giving birth. Surely you would prefer to see these events through, even if you were in pain, rather than not at all.

Let me give an example from my own company. We recently introduced in the United States a product for a disease known in France as Maladie de Charcot, known elsewhere Motor Neuron Disease, ALS or Lou Gehrig's disease. I will come back to this product more later on but I would like to quote to you a poem sent in to us by a patient when we introduced the product via the Internet.

"Love We Hold"

Don't take one day for granted - For we have no guarantee
That we'll get all we've wanted - Or live to ninety-three
Don't take one breath for granted - I'd like you all to see
That all we've ever needed-Lives inside of you and me
Each day is but a wonder-Such beauty to behold
It is nothing but pure blunder - Not to harvest each day's gold
Being in the present - Not the future or the past
Living out each moment - is the way to make them last
The only reason that we live - Or so my heart's been told
is to learn how to give - And to cherish the love we hold.

Which brings us to one of the major problems of assessment. Quality of life is not just a matter of objective tests, but also a matter of subjective judgment as has been brought out clearly during this conference.

A study by Jachuck published in 1982 asked doctors, patients and patients' close companions whether patients' conditions improved, worsened or remained unchanged after treatment by anti-hypertensive agents.

All the doctors thought their patients had improved. By contrast, only 48% of the patients felt they had improved and 8% thought they were worse off. Most strikingly, nearly all the relatives felt that the patients were worse, with many reporting impairment of memory, irritability, lack of energy and decline in sexual interest. Not problems that are readily discerned in a 15 minute interview.

Ten years later an article by Slevin in the British Medical Journal stated very bluntly that: "doctors and nurses are notoriously unreliable at estimating patients' quality of life."

In all fairness to the doctors, patients make mistakes too. It is not uncommon for patients to confuse side-effects of the treatment with the disease itself.

The fact is that problems are there to be overcome. Nobody knows better than the medical profession that it takes a long time to initiate and carry through major advances. At the moment, it is clear that data gained from quality of life assessments are often not adequately "hard" to use as a basis for decisions. But in time they will improve. After all, the clinical trials of the 1960's are nothing compared to those our industry regularly performs today. This refinement took time and so too will quality of life measurement.

Whilst I am not the greatest fan of the late Chairman Mao, I applaud his concept of letting a thousand flowers bloom, especially if they can bloom without having the heads cut off.

I am therefore delighted, when I read from learned journals, to see the growing number of systems for assessing the quality of life.

We have the Functional Living Index for Cancer; the Spitzer Quality of Life Index; the European Organization for Research and Treatment of Cancer Care Quality and the Cancer Rehabilitations System - Short Form. And others besides. One of the best is called Q-TWIST which stands for Quality-Adjusted Time Without Symptoms of Disease and Toxicity of Treatment.

However many believe that today the best method for assessing the key medical dimensions of quality of life for cancer patient remains the Rotterdam Symptom Checklist. It takes about 8 minutes of interview, is easy to score and is divided into two main subscales, one for physical complaints and one for psychological issues. We need to get feedback directly from the patient and his or her family.

My hope is that before long we can gather in the "thousand blooms" from these various systems to be able to reach a consensus judgment on the value of treatment options, including palliative care.

Hopefully there will be outside pressures from doctors, patient groups and government officials to agree on the applicability of quality of life scores within the different cancer treatments. We will then have established a proxy for value in this area.

2. WELL-SATISFIED AND UNSATISFIED TREATMENT AREAS

When at last we arrive at sound proxies for value in the use of medicines, how should we use them in resource allocation? Let me look at two groups of diseases and see if value measurements can have the same meaning in resource allocation decisions.

Hypertension is an example of a disease which is generally well-satisfied. If a new medicine comes along now, quality of life measurement will indeed have a place in assessing how much money health systems are prepared to pay for it. If the gain in quality is 10% then why not pay 10% more? It is difficult to deny the logic in this.

Well-satisfied disease areas are not, however, the subject of our meeting. No one can be satisfied with the current treatment of cancer, of AIDS or of a myriad of other serious conditions.

Among cancer types few are well treated and even those that are could benefit from more patient-friendly medicines. If a new drug were produced for breast, lung or colon cancers, areas my company among others is deeply involved with, what would be the impact of tying price rigidly to the improvement in efficacy and quality of life?

In answering this question, history should be our guide. There has been no "magic bullet" for any cancer type, each advance has been incremental. Gene therapy, which RPR is very much involved with, may result in true cures, possibly even prevention. While gene therapy holds out many promises, its progress may well be step-by-step. If the taxoids are an advance over platinum, then a p53 gene/retrovirus combination could be a major step, and a p53 gene/adenovirus construct could be a useful incremental improvement.

So, if the first step in gene therapy were 10% better than the existing treatment, and the next two steps 10% better again, should they be priced accordingly? Strict following of the doctrine of quality of life measurement would imply that they should. Yet were this to happen, what would be the impact on research, or medical advances, and the quality of life of patients in the future? The answer is simple. It would stamp out the vital first steps of progress which are the beginning of the road to a well-satisfied disease area. Without those first steps there can be no progress. Pharmaceutical companies could not afford to take the higher risk, higher cost research for an innovative "first step" product if the price were going to be tied to what is likely to be a modest improvement.

It was Neil Armstrong who took "One small step for man" and "one giant leap for mankind". That first step on the moon was not subject to some sort of economic micro-measurement; it was done because of what it meant to mankind - or at least to the U.S.!

Medical advances are rarely so dramatic. I referred earlier to the launch of a new medicine in the USA which brings an average of three months increase in patients life expectancy, and little impact on the quality of that life. The disease is Maladie de Charcot, or ALS. The medicine, Rilutek®, is the first one to be approved for treatment of this disease since it was first described over 120 years ago. Such a medicine is clearly not the end of development in this disease. But it is the first step.

To price such a product by its efficacy or its quality of life impact only would be to declare that innovation itself is largely worthless - in which case patients could be condemned to no treatment for a further 120 years perhaps. That is not a message I for one would like to deliver to the 1,200 people, mostly patients, who joined our U.S. Rilutek conference on the Internet last week.

We simply cannot compare the value - added in a disease area where other successful treatment options exist with the value - added in diseases where they do not.

3. CAUTION

"A little learning is a dangerous thing", and never has this been more true than in medicines. Quality of life data are simply not yet adequate to make resource allocation decisions, particularly for diseases like cancer and AIDS. And anyone who tries to do so, will sound warning bells among those committed to innovation for patient benefit, whatever our profession.

Let me refer briefly to a recent debate in the United Kingdom over the use of beta-inteferon for use in multiple sclerosis. Before this product was approved, the UK National Health Service Executive prepared guidelines advising that this innovative - and expensive - first step product be reserved for consultants to prescribe only.

This guidance led to a debate about the rationing of health care. While the word "rationing" was rejected by the British Health Secretary, he did say that there must be more rigorous scrutiny of what treatments the NHS paid for - so-called "evidence based medicine." Were this comment to be applied to minor treatments such as some cosmetic surgeries, there would be little cause for concern. But that is not all that is involved.

The British doctors' organization, the Royal College of Physicians recently produced a report called "Setting Priorities in the NHS: A Framework for Decision-making.", calling for more public debate about the issue of health rationing in Britain. But in calling for a debate that report could help to bring forward rationing itself. One of the report's sections was reported as saying that *"when it is thought necessary to deny funds for effective but costly treatments and investigations,* there should be an agreed procedure to help doctors...". The Royal College of Physicians report is thus inherently accepting that effective but costly treatments should be withheld. How frightening! Events such as these, along with the widespread underuse of expensive products such as thrombolytics, erythropoietin and Pulmozyme, give me great concern about the impact budgetary constraint is having on quality of care in the country of my birth.

When seeking to control budgets it is always seductive to find "independent" support for ones decisions. Throughout history, good ideas have been used to mask questionable ambitions. If anyone were to say that a really innovative medicine in an area where treatment was unsatisfactory was not worth an innovation premium they should not be allowed to hide behind quality of life measures. Their motive should be clear to all - budget control not patient benefit.

CONCLUSION

Today, the status of quality of life measurements is similar to that of clinical trials of my youth - imperfect, developing rapidly, but at the same time all that we have. Such measurements, properly used, should be encouraged. They should not be pressed into the service of budget-cutting ends for which they are as yet ill-suited and, more dangerously, could lead to discontinuing or discrediting what are otherwise important developments.

In serious disease where treatment is not yet satisfactory, like AIDS, cancer or Maladie de Charcot, innovative medicine prices should not be tied to quality of life scores. To do so would discourage research progress, as incremental gains often occur at exponential extra cost. But without the encouragement of initial gains, major progress will not happen.

In short, the valuation of innovation in AIDS, cancer and other serious diseases is too important to be left solely in the hands of the economist, even of the distinguished health economists we have heard from at this Congress.

CONCLUSION

Harvey V. Fineberg

Harvard School of Public Health
677 Huntington Ave.
Boston, Massachusetts 02115

All who come to a conference like this bring our own experience, our own background and our perspective on the questions that we are discussing. Inevitably, each of us will take away a personal picture enriched by the insights of others and yet different in the end from any other because of what we each brought to such a gathering.

Two of the most ancient precepts of western medicine are first, do no harm, and second, do all you can to preserve the life of your patient. In modern medicine, and particularly in the experience with cancer, AIDS and other serious diseases, these ancient precepts have demanded reexamination. In treating cancer, for example, the clinician often takes calculated risks by imposing difficult treatments, disfiguring treatments, painful treatments, treatments that test the patient and the family, for the purpose and with the hope of achieving a better result in the end. The physician is willing to do harm at first to achieve a greater benefit in the long term. Also, because of advances in medical technology for treating many conditions that previously reached a terminal stage, we now have the capacity to sustain life beyond the time when it may be meaningful life to live. So the old precepts to do no harm and at all costs to sustain life no longer hold in an unqualified way. This recognition brings us to the motivating question behind this symposium: How can we accommodate the quality of life as a guide and a goal in the care of individual patients and as a purpose in society?

Today we must also face squarely the cost of care. We have heard many eloquent statements in the course of this meeting to the effect that it is essential for any beneficial treatment to be made available to a patient. At the same time, we have been told that it is necessary to use available resources wisely in the care of all patients, to benefit all of society. The economists constantly remind us that it is not possible simultaneously to achieve the greatest productivity and good while spending the least amount possible. These are incompatible objectives. So, how do we reconcile the desire to do everything we are able to do for the benefit of patients, with the compulsion to control our resources and to use them to benefit all of the public?

These conflicting objectives also motivate the search for some way of judging the value of medical interventions. This, in turn, requires a capacity to find measures that reflect the quality of life to help guide expenditures on practices that work and that worthwhile.

Cancer, AIDS, and Quality of Life, edited by Levy *et al.*
Plenum Press, New York, 1997

We went on, in the course of this meeting, to confront a fundamental dilemma. The imperatives of modern medicine and technical capacity, the exigencies of chronic diseases like cancer and AIDS, the pressure of constrained resources, all lead us to seek measures for the quality of life. Yet, at the same time, as speaker after speaker has reflected on the meaning of the quality of life and on the utility of quality of life measures as related to health, we have heard one after another express mild to grave reservations about our capacity to measure and represent the quality of life. In other words, we must assess the quality of life, yet we cannot be confident in our ability to do so.

If there has been a dominant, underlying principle expressed by those who spoke at this conference, it is that the quality of life ultimately resides in the personal, subjective, individual perception of each individual, and that perception must in turn be conditioned by experience and culture. The idea that the patient in the medical context is the origin, and should be the only legitimate origin, of judgments about quality of life was perhaps the most pervasive theme throughout the several days of our meeting. We were reminded that the quality of life is not synonymous with the quality of health and that the quality of health, in turn, is not equal to the quality of medical care. We must be wary, as speaker after speaker alerted us, to confusing what we are doing in medicine, what we are achieving in health, and what we are attempting as a society to attain for every citizen, a better quality of life. So let us be careful as we proceed from this conference to focus the available measures of quality of life on the particular purposes for which we are applying such measures. Let us not deceive ourselves or others about the relation between what we measure in medicine and health and what we are trying to achieve in each person and in society.

Our conference revealed a number of core values and philosophic principles widely shared by those who spoke. The most central perhaps is the principle of humanism, of confidence in the individual value and dignity of human life, of elevating that value above all others. There was a pervasive sense of what I would describe as anti-authoritarianism in the presentations. This is reflected in the desire to gain from each individual a personal, independent assessment of what is right for that individual, and of repeated calls on the medical profession to seek out and respect the desires of the patient. We heard especially from the contributions of those from parts of Africa, outside of western Europe or North America, the value of communitarianism, the idea of the interdependence of the individual's sense of self-worth on the support and love of the family and community in which each of us resides.

We began our conference with what might be considered the fundamental, contemporary scientific dialectic: the alternative pathways to progress in science through reductionism on the one side versus holism on the other. Most of what we do in western science depends upon a reductionist philosophy of breaking down complicated problems into their constituent parts. We seek to understand the mechanisms of each of the constituents and search for the linkages and ways in which those elemental constituents add up to the totality. An alternative approach in biological and other sciences attempts to apprehend the whole of the subject and experience. This is particularly relevant to the discussions that we had about approaches to trying to assess and learn about the quality of life as perceived by each individual.

My own feeling is that perhaps we understated the importance of focusing on the particular purposes for which one is attempting to proceed with measures like quality of life. We considered, for example, looking at health-related quality of life as a means toward establishing a philosophy and an approach to health care through our discussions about palliative and curative services. We engaged in much discussion about the purpose of looking at quality of life in the evaluation of clinical care: enabling better decisions between doctor and patient, judging what interventions (pharmaceutical, surgical or other) work or do not work, and gauging the ultimate benefit of medical services. Third, we sometimes talked about the purpose of allocating resources in a society that has many more opportunities to expend resources with possible benefits, than it has resources available to expend. And finally, although we did not spend much time on it, we could think about measures of quality of life such as those introduced by the World Health Organization and others as means toward achieving a kind of global index of well-being analogous to the economic measure of net national product, providing a way to compare from one country to another the quality of life experienced by individuals in each society.

Each of these purposes—setting a philosophy of care, evaluating services, allocating resources or creating an index of well-being—brings with it a set of difficulties and concerns about the appropriateness of measurement, the nature of measurement, the ways in which measures can be interpreted and utilized for making decisions. During this symposium, we have considered the reasons why we should attempt to measure quality of life and some of the strengths of these efforts. We have also weighed these reasons and strengths against the limitations of such measures and our concerns and misgivings about their use.

I would like to conclude by offering three reflections prompted by our discussion at the symposium. First, regardless of how well we can measure quality of life, it is inevitable that implicitly or explicitly we will be taking account of quality of life in our judgments about care of individual patients and use of health resources. We cannot escape the reality that length of life is no longer a sufficient basis for making individual decisions or spending social resources. What we can ask ourselves, however, is whether it is better to act in a kind of knowing ignorance of the measure of quality of life or whether we should make a pretense of knowing more than we actually can know at a time when we must make decisions. Neither is a very attractive alternative, and I think the task for us is to select and validate, and with a high degree of humility, apply the measures we can to the particular needs.

Second, I believe, perhaps as an inveterate optimist, that it is possible for us to make progress in our use of measures of quality of life and that their application can improve decisions on the part of individual patients and on the part of society. I believe it is possible to do so, as long as we do not overstate what we know at any point in time. We have talked about the fact that there are now numerous measures available. To those who are engaged in the practice of using these and evaluating them, I urge, carry on that work. We need the results of your labors. We need to have more reliable and certified ways of guiding decisions. In the end, however, we must know that these decisions cannot rest entirely on such imperfect measures of quality. Ultimately, the decisions will depend on the judgment of patients, doctors, policy makers, people in the judicial system, scientists, journalists—indeed everyone who plays a part in the political process—to make wise decisions based on what we know at the time we must make those decisions.

And finally, I would say that if any point has come repeatedly to the fore in these discussions, it has been the importance and the value of honest and open communication at all levels: between patients and their caregivers, communicating in both directions, and in the public's participation in the democratic process, contributing to decisions about resource use and priorities. In the end, the decisions that are made will affect everyone, and each individual has a right to participate in those decisions. Taking better advantage of the new technologies available electronically and by other means, to open these channels of communication holds great promise. In my opinion we can never hope to find a superior substitute for the open heart of individuals seeking honestly to learn from and to share with one another. This perhaps is the ultimate lesson from our symposium.

In closing, I would like to express my appreciation to the supporters and organizers of the symposium and especially to Jay Levy and to Gabriel Bez, who together worked so hard in organizing the scientific program, and most of all, to Claude Jasmin, whose efforts made it possible for us to gather in this way. Thank you very much.

INDEX

Achievement–aspiration relationship, 46–48, 49, 50
Acquired immunodeficiency syndrome (AIDS)
  comparison with cancer, 18–20
  immune system in, 17, 18, 19–20, 24–25
  incurability of, 173
  pathogenesis of, 18–20
  symptoms of, 19–20, 29
  treatment of
    clinical trials of, 180
    in developing countries, 170–172
    of opportunistic infections, 9
  United Nations Joint Programme on HIV/AIDS
    (UNAIDS), 7–10
Acquired immunodeficiency syndrome epidemic: see
  Human immunodeficiency virus infection
  (HIV)/AIDS epidemic
Acquired immunodeficiency syndrome (AIDS) patients
  activism of, 1–2, 3, 151–152
  attitudes towards quality of life questionnaires of,
    157
  discrimination towards, 8, 152, 172
  family members of, 7, 10, 145, 146
  medical caregivers of, 133–134
  participation in health care decision-making, 115
  quality of health care for, 170–172
  quality of life of, 64–66, 70
  stigmatization of, 141, 143, 144–145, 146, 152, 157,
    172
Activities of daily living impairments (ADLIs), of
  AIDS patients, 66
Advocacy, see also Activism
  for cancer patients, 101–105
Affective disorders, in cancer patients, 73–75
Africa
  HIV/AIDS epidemic in, 141–142
    family-based care system for, 145
    impact on women, 145, 146
    patient care in, 143, 144, 145
    stigmatization of AIDS patients in, 144–145,
      146
  tradition of solidarity in, 124–125
Age factors, in quality of life, 121
Antiretroviral drugs, as AIDS treatment, 2, 9, 21, 171

Anxiety
  of cancer patients, 73
  of terminally-ill patients, 90
Association of the Ladies of Calvary, 132, 164, 165

Biologic reductionism, 12, 14
Biomedical cure, of disease, 150, 151
Bone marrow transplantation, 24, 78, 79, 80
Brain, see also Psychoneuroimmunology
  relationship with gastrointestinal system, 26
Breast cancer
  genetic screening for, 19, 22, 108, 109, 174–175
  treatment of
    cost-efficiency of, 78, 79
    quality of life considerations in, 69

Cancer
  diagnosis of
    disclosure to patient, 73–75, 98–100, 131, 90
    genetic screening and, 107–109
    patient's psychological adjustment to, 73–75
  genetic testing for, 3, 17, 18, 22, 173–177
  immune system in, 17, 18, 19–20, 24–25
  incurability of, 132, 132–133, 163, 164–165, 173
  pathogenesis of, 18–20
  quality of life measures for, 185
  risk status determination in, 107–113
  treatment of, 97, 185–186
    basic research in, 2, 17–18, 20–21
    immunotherapy, 24–25
    palliative treatment, 2, 92–93, 97, 131, 132
    toxicity of, 18, 20, 23–24
Cancer patients
  advocacy for, 101–105
  associations of, 165–166
  educational level of, 99–100
  genetic counseling of, 101–105
  medical caregivers for, 133–135
  quality of life of, 163–167
    affective disorders and, 73–75
    questionnaire assessment of, 3
Cancer Rehabilitations System-Short Form, 185
CASPER mnemonic, for quality of life, 42

CD4$^+$ cells, opiate-like substance production by, 27
CD8$^+$ cells, use in immunotherapy, 24
Cervical cancer, genetic screening for, 22, 108
Chemotherapy
    quality of life considerations in, 185–186
    toxicity of, 18, 20, 23–24, 189
China, quality of life assessment in, 161
Clinical trials, 180–181
    quality of life criterion for, 3, 69
Clinton administration, health care plan of, 57–58, 59
Colon cancer
    cost-utility evaluation of, 78, 79
    genetic screening for, 22, 108, 174
Community, role in HIV/AIDS epidemic, 145,
        151–152, 190
Conditioned stimuli, therapeutic use of, 28–29
Consent, of patient, for end-of-life care, 123–124
Consumerisn, in health care, 56, 57, 103
Counseling
    of AIDS patients, 8
    genetic, of cancer patients, 101–105
Cultural bias, of quality of life measures, 155–157, 158
Cytokines
    as fatigue cause, 27
    production of
        in AIDS and cancer, 19–20, 22
        by nervous, endocrine, and immune systems,
            19–20, 22, 25, 26
    therapeutic use of, 2, 24–25, 30

Death and dying, 92, 133, 137–140
    dignity in, 93, 97, 123
    peaceful, 46, 93–95
    physicians' attitudes towards, 89–93, 129–130
    prognosis of, 139–140
    quality of life and, 119–127
Disabled persons, quality of life of, 11, 156
Discrimination, towards HIV/AIDS patients, 8, 152,
        172
Drug therapy, 183–187; see also Chemotherapy;
        names of specific drugs

Ecology metaphor, of health care, 58–60, 61
Economic evaluation, of cancer and AIDS treatment,
        77–84
    cost/quality adjusted life years (QALY) measure,
        78, 79, 80–81, 83–84
    cost/quality of life related to time without symp-
        toms and toxicity (Q-TWIST) measure, 78,
        81–83, 185
    cost/years of life gained measure, 78
European Organization for Research and Treatment of
        Cancer Care Quality (EORTC), 64, 185
EuroQol (quality of life measure), 64
Euthanasia, 4, 130, 140
    physician's role in, 94, 124, 129

Functional Living Index for Cancer, 185

Genetic screening, predictive, 3–4, 19, 22, 173–177

Genetic screening, predictive (cont.)
    counseling associated with, 101–105
    risk diagnosis in, 3, 107–113
Global Domestic Product (GDP), relationship to
        health status, 148, 149, 150
Greece, ancient
    physicians' attitudes towards death in, 90
    quality of life concept in, 38

Health
    concept of, 109–112
    definition of, 77, 110, 170
    relationship to quality of life, 42, 156, 157
    relationship to socioeconomic status, 148–150
Health care
    consumerism in, 56, 57, 103
    equitable access to, by AIDS patients, 157–158
    gender discrimination in, 144
    preventive, 6, 59–60, 176
    resource allocation in, 69–70, 145, 187, 189, 190,
        191
Health care costs, effect on health care delivery effec-
        tiveness, 77–84
    cost/quality adjusted life year (QALY) measure 78,
        79, 80–81, 83–84
    cost/quality of life relationship to time without
        symptoms and toxicity (Q-TWIST) measure,
        78, 81–83
    cost/year of life gained measure, 78
Health care reform
    Clinton administration plan for, 57–58, 59
    main issues in, 150–151
Health insurance companies
    genetic screening information use by, 175–176
    market approach to health coverage by, 56–57
Hormones, production by neuro-endocrine-immune
        system, 25
Hospice movement, 91, 131, 132, 165
Human genome research, 60, 173–178
    implication for drug development, 176–177
    predictive genetic tests, 3–4, 19, 22, 173–177
        counseling associated with, 101–105
        risk diagnosis in, 107–113
Human immunodeficiency virus (HIV) infection
    in Africa
        family-based care system for, 145
        impact on women, 145, 146
        patient care in, 143, 144, 145
        stigmatization of patients in, 144–145, 146
    age factors in, 171
    antibody testing, 3, 8
    early detection of, 22–23
    latency of, 19
    opportunistic infections of, 171
    treatment of
        antiretroval therapy, 2, 9, 21, 171
        basic research in, 17–18, 21
        immunotherapy, 24–25
        quality of care in, 170–172
        in developing countries, 169–172

Immune response
   in cancer and AIDS, 17, 19–20
      enhancement of, 18, 24–25
      sensory function of, 28
Immunotherapy, 24–25
Income per capita, in developing countries, 169–170

Laparoscopy patients, risk-adjusted functional status
      of, 86
Leukemia
   bone marrow transplants and, 19, 20–21
   medical decision-making regarding, 116–117
Life expectancy
   during eighteenth century, 130
   increase of, 89, 129, 149–150
   effect of medical treatment on, 89
   as quality of life measure, 184
Life-sustaining techniques, 129–130
   discontinuation of, 138
   effect of quality of life, 189
Living wills, 123, 125, 138
Lymphocytes
   receptors on, 26, 27
   stress-induced proliferation of, 28

Managed care, 56–57
Market metaphor, of health care, 55, 56–57, 60
Military metaphor, of health care, 55, 56, 60

Neuropeptides, 25–26, 27, 30

Pain
   experienced by dying patients, 137
   management of
      inadequacy of, 2, 9
      in palliative care, 125
Palliative care
   for AIDS patients, 9
   for cancer patients, 2, 92–93, 97, 131, 132
   outcome of, 45, 50–52
   patient's knowledge of terminal status and,
      123–124
   quality of life during, 121
Patient associations
   of AIDS patients, 1, 3, 166
   of cancer patients, 165–166
Pharmaceutical industry, cancer and AIDS drug treat-
      ment research by, 179–181
Physician-patient relationship, of terminally-ill pa-
      tients, 89–91, 98, 121–127, 134, 137–138
   of disadvantaged patients, 134
   disclosure in, 98, 123–124
Preventive health care, 176
   ecological approach in, 59–60
Prostate cancer
   early detection of, 22
   quality of life in, 67, 86–87
   treatment of, adverse effects of, 17, 86

Psychological aspects, of quality of life, 122, 159–
      160
Psychoneuroimmunology, 18, 25–29, 30, 112
Public health care
   in AIDS epidemic, 1, 152
   developing countries' lack of, 170
   ecological approach of, 59–60

Quality-adjusted life years (QALY), 78, 79, 80–81,
      83–84, 116
Quality of care
   health model of, 142–143
   effect of quality of life on, 49–53
      care outcome, 45, 50–52
      for HIV/AIDS patients, 170–172
      philosophy of care and, 49, 50–51, 53
      resource availability and, 52–53
Quality of life
   of AIDS patients, maximization of, 8–10
   aspiration-achievement gap measure of, 46–48, 49, 50
   of cancer patients, 3, 73–75, 163–167
   components of, 119–121
   cultural aspect, 141–146, 161
      versus medical aspect, 142–144
   definition of, 2, 37, 112, 119–120, 147–148
   geographic aspect of, 141, 161
   health-related, 37, 63–72, 190
      of AIDS patients, 64–66, 70
      measurement, 63–72
   medically conceptualized, 142–144, 145, 146
   personal nature of, 120–121, 190
   physical, 39, 46, 47
   psychological aspects of, 122, 159–160
   relationship to clinical care, 190–191
   relationship to health, 2, 11, 14, 109, 190
   socio-economic aspect of, 141–153
Quality of life measures, 190
   cultural bias of, 155–157, 158
   deficiencies in, 11–15
   use in drug therapy, 183–187
   ethnocentricity of, 155–157
   health-related, 63–72, 85–88, 156
   medical orientation of, 155–158
   statistical reductionism in, 11, 12–14
Quality of life related to time without symptoms and
      toxicity (Q-TWIST), 78, 81–83
Quantity of life, 122

Reductionism, 12–14
Religious aspect, of quality of life, 5, 42, 46, 48, 120,
      156–157, 159–160
Resource allocation, in health care, 69–70, 145, 189,
      190, 191
Risk
   as diagnosis, 107–113
   illness-disease-sickness relationship of, 111–112

Short Form-36 Physical Function Index (SIP), 64, 86

Socio-economic factors
  in health, 148–150
  in HIV/AIDS epidemic, 151
  in quality of life, 147–153
Stigmatization, of HIV/AIDS patients, 141, 143,
      144–145, 146, 152, 157, 172
Structural adjustment policies (SAPs), 169
Study to Understand Prognoses and Preferences for
      Outcomes and Risks of Treatment (SUP-
      PORT), 137–140
Suicide
  physician-assisted, 94, 124, 129
  rational, 94
SUPPORT (Study to Understand Prognoses and Prefer-
      ences for Outcomes and Risks of Treat-
      ment), 137–140
Support Team Assessment Schedule, 52

T cells, 24, 26
United Kingdom
  health care rationing in, 187
  hospice movement in, 91, 131, 132
  Pain Society of, 2
United Nations Joint Programme on HIV/AIDS
      (UNAIDS), 7–10
Universal Declaration of Human Rights, 97

Women
  impact of HIV/AIDS epidemic on, 145, 146
  powerlessness of, 5
World Health Organization (WHO)
  cancer pain treatment recommendation of, 131
  health definition of, 77
  Quality of Life Assessment (WHOQOL) question-
      naire, 159–162, 170

INTERNATIONAL COUNCIL FOR GLOBAL HEALTH PROGRESS

Despite recent scientific progress against disease, health remains a major concern for every nation on earth. Health care systems in all countries are finding it increasingly difficult to cope with rapidly changing events of a medical nature, and their social and economic sequelae. A new vision of global health is clearly necessary. It is the mission of the International Council for Global Health Progress (ICGHP) to contribute to this new approach and to confront its inherent challenges.

The International Council for Global Health Progress is a non-profit, interdisciplinary organization founded in 1992. Its major objective is to fashion a scientific approach to the assessment of health needs, and to the delineation of possible solutions to current, as well as potential, health issues. The Council is independent of all government and international health agencies. Since its inception, the ICGHP has been studying health issues of a worldwide nature and making recommendations for appropriate approaches. In achieving its objectives, the ICGHP has the following specific aims:

- to create think-tanks, training programs and educational initiatives.
- to organize international conferences characterized by a global approach and top-level participants.
- to share its findings with the appropriate national and international organizations.

ADMINISTRATION

Executive Committee

Claude Jasmin, M.D., F.A.C.P. - President
  Professor of Oncology,
  Chairman, Department of Hematology, Immunology and Biology,
  Hopital Paul Brousse, Villejuif, France
Harvey V. Fineberg, M.D., Ph.D. - Vice-President
  Dean, Harvard School of Public Health, Boston
Gordon, J. Piller, O.B.E., Ph.D., F.R.C.P. -Treasurer
  Founder and former Director of the Leukemia Research Fund, London
  Member, Universities of London and Leeds

Board of Directors

Elena Androunas, Ph.D.
   Director, COMCON, Communication Consulting Co. Moscow
Gabriel Bez
   Director, "Mission SIDA", French Ministry of Health, Paris
Robert N. Butler, M.D.
   Professor of Gerontology and Geriatrics, Mount Sinai Medical Center
   Director, International Longevity Center, New York
   Pulitzer Prize Winner
Lawrence K. Grossman
   President, Horizons TV
   Former President, NBC News
Noelle Lenoir
   Member of the Constitutional Council
   Chair, UNESCO Bioethics Advisory Committee
   Chair, Advisors on the Ethical Implications of Biotechnology,
   European Commission
Jay A. Levy, M.D.
   Professor of Medicine,
   Research Associate, Cancer Research Institute,
   University of California School of Medicine, San Francisco
Eva Nowotny, Ph.D.
   Austrian Ambassador to England
Kihumbu Thairu, M.B ChB
   Professor of Medicine,
   Medical Advisor and Director of Health Program,
   Commonwealth Regional Secretariat, Arusha, Kenya
   Former Dean, Faculty of Medicine, University of Nairobi
Elie Wiesel
   Professor of Philosphy, Boston University, Boston
   Author, Winner of the 1986 Nobel Peace Prize

Consultant in International Relations

Peter H. Berczeller, M.D., F.A.C.P.
   Professor of Clinical Medicine,
   New York University School of Medicine, New York